Nursing:
The Practice of Caring

Nursing:
The Practice of Caring

Anne H. Bishop and John R. Scudder, Jr.

National League for Nursing Press • New York
Pub. No. 14-2442

Copyright © 1991
National League for Nursing
350 Hudson Street, New York, NY 10014

ISBN 0-88737-537-5

The views expressed in this book reflect those of the authors and do not necessarily reflect the official views of the National League for Nursing.

This book was set in Goudy by Publications Development Company. The editor and designer was Allan Graubard. Northeastern Press was the printer and binder. The cover was designed by Lillian Welsh.

Printed in the United States of America.

Dedication

To Millie and Irv

Friends who taught us the importance of giving and receiving care while living in the face of terminal illness.

About the Authors

Anne H. Bishop, EdD, RN, is Professor, Department of Nursing, Lynchburg College, Lynchburg, Virginia.

John R. Scudder, Jr., PhD, is Professor of Philosophy and Education, Lynchburg College, Lynchburg, Virginia.

Contents

Foreword

Anne H. Bishop and John R. Scudder, Jr. have provided here a wonderful introduction to what it means to take a practicalist turn in philosophy and, in the process, have given seriousness and meaning to notions of good embedded in the caring practice of nursing. They are to be commended for a readable work based on strong philosophical underpinnings. This book is especially worth reading if for no other clarification than that between the confusing and unpromising debate between craft-oriented "workers" and scientific technicians. While the first group is comprised of traditionalists, the second group directs technology through science with neither having a critical or ethical stance by which to guide and evaluate technology. Faced with this cul de sac, Bishop and Scudder call on the nursing profession to transcend both technological self-understandings, without, at the same time, denigrating technology designed to provide humane care and effective cures. Other important clarifications and discussions also make this book worth thoughtful reading and debate—a highly effective medium for discussions in issues and trends classes as well as theory and philosophy courses in nursing.

Significantly, this book represents an important turn in ethical discourse that takes the reader beyond Kantian-based procedural ethics to consider the notions of good embedded in excellent nursing practice. Such thoughtful study of practice forms the basis for understanding everyday relational ethics and leads to thinking and theorizing about the discipline of nursing. In so doing, the authors call attention to the post-critical philosophical turn to practice in order to address the limits of formal theoretical knowledge, and the loss of a shared language outside of practice for making distinctions of worth. These problems, the authors contend, are addressed in narratives of excellent practice as provided. Clinicians will find encouragement and vision in this book.

Bishop and Scudder call on the feminist writings of Gilligan and Noddings on caring to address the ethics embedded in a caring practice. Here they clearly take a liberation stance clarifying that "In a philosophy of practice, excellent practice does not mean merely continuing current practice, however competently, but obligates practitioners to reform that practice and expand its legitimate authority whenever fostering patient well being requires it." They clarify that caring practice is not a sentimental, internal feeling but a skilled technique imbued with knowledge and notions of good. While the place of caring in nursing is sometimes feared to be the source of status inequity and subservience, this work demonstrates that we dare not abandon our caring practices. To do so may purchase some negative "freedom from" but, in the process, almost surely will cause nursing to lose the positive freedom that gives it its voice and its power to heal, cure, foster health, and provide comfort.

Finally, this book adds an important voice to the current debates about curriculum reform in nursing education. Any faculty member considering course and curricular design will do well to consider this work as a thoughtful exploration of redesigning nursing education to more closely meet the demands of excellent nursing practice.

Patricia Benner, PhD, RN, FAAN
Professor
Department of Physiological Nursing
University of California
San Francisco, California

1

Phenomenological Interpretation of Nursing

During the past several years, nurse educators have sought to redefine their role and that of nursing in the ever changing world of health care. Advocates of the new curriculum, for example, have even proclaimed the need for revolution in nurse education (Moccia, 1990), rooting their work in a distinctive reinterpretation of the meaning of nursing itself. Unlike other reformative strategies in nursing education that measure success or failure in terms of keeping pace with scientific and technological changes, this revolution finds its strength and purpose in the act of caring. As such, attempts to reformulate nursing and nursing education as sciences and technologies are severely criticized. Although the attempt to subsume human practices under the logic and language of scientific technology so common in our time is questionable, it is a particularly grave mistake when considering the practice of caring. Critical appraisal of scientific and technological institutions is not lim-ited to questioning their appropriateness for a caring practice but also appraises the very meaning in which these institutions are rooted. For nursing, the effects of such questioning of essential roots focuses on its fundamental meaning and future shape: Will nursing continue to be reconstituted as an applied science or will its reinterpretation as a caring practice be fully realized?

The answer to the question above depends on meanings ascribed to caring and practice and to science and technology and how their interrelationships are seen. Phenomenological interpretation, the philosophical methodology that seeks to disclose essential meanings as encountered in the lived world, offers a particularly productive way of exploring the meaning of nursing. Although much attention in nursing has been focused on doing rather than meaning, for the profession to mature it is now imperative to consider the essential meaning of nursing itself.

Much of the present confusion concerning the meaning of nursing comes from the definition of the word; *nursing* refers both to care for patients and to the study of that care. In the nursing literature, these two senses of nursing are often confused. For example, those who regard nursing as a science often mean that nursing is best studied scientifically, rather than that nursing care itself is a science. Although much can be learned from the scientific study of nursing, the assertion that it is best studied scientifically is surely debatable. Certainly, it is even more questionable that the practice of nursing itself is a science. The inadequacy of the latter contention is made evident by making a clear distinction between nursing as a practice and nursing as a discipline. Thus, for this book, we will designate the study of nursing as the discipline of nursing to distinguish it from the practice of nursing.

NURSING AS DISCIPLINE AND AS PRACTICE

To clarify the distinction between nursing as a practice and nursing as a discipline and to introduce phenomenological interpretation, we offer a phenomenological interpretation of the following example.

Berit, a nurse who was a graduate student in education in a European university, presented her first paper at an international human science conference. She was understandably nervous since the audience was made up mostly of established scholars. However, Berit confidently presented her argument that nursing is a science because she anticipated that this audience of human science scholars would be in sympathy with her position. Consequently, she was perplexed when an established nursing scholar, Susan, challenged her position by arguing that nursing is neither a science nor an applied science but a practice. During the discussion that continued after the session, Susan was able to discuss with Berit more fully her thesis that nursing is a practice that should be studied by the human sciences.

At the next annual conference, when Susan presented a paper, a young woman in the audience asked some very excellent questions. When Susan and the young woman continued their discussion after the session, the young woman mentioned the sharpness of the criticism with which Susan had responded to her paper at the previous year's conference. It was only then that Susan recognized Berit. She apologized for the harshness of her criticism and explained that at the time of the previous conference she was preoccupied with the thesis of her new book that nursing is a practice and not a science or applied science and that nursing should be studied by using phenomenological interpretation.

Berit responded that the criticism had been justified and that it had helped her to redirect her thought in a way that had contributed to the dissertation she was working on in her country. Susan admitted that she, too, had once thought that nursing should be studied as a science when, some years ago, she moved from a hospital to a collegiate setting. At that time she regarded science merely as a systematic way of understanding nursing which also would supplant the popular view that nursing primarily consisted of practical methodology. Berit asked Susan what had changed her mind. Susan responded that she had encountered phenomenological interpretation and saw in it a way of articulating the meaning of nursing that would make sense both to the academic community and to practicing nurses.

When the example above is interpreted in light of the recent history of nursing education, the confusion resulting from the failure to distinguish between the practice of nursing and the discipline of nursing comes sharply into focus. Like many nurses who suddenly found themselves in an academic setting, Berit and Susan had initially wanted to articulate nursing as a science, but neither had given much thought to the meaning of science. It also is apparent that neither had given much thought to the distinction between nursing as an academic discipline and nursing as practiced.

Berit's and Susan's discussions make the need for this distinction very evident. When Berit contended, as Susan once believed, that nursing should be a science, she really was contending that the discipline of nursing should be a science. Having been a practicing nurse, she certainly was not arguing that nursing care was constituted as a science. At most, certain procedures used in nursing practice could be described as applied science, but this certainly does not mean that nursing care, as a whole, can be constituted as an applied science. It is easy for professors and others engaged in nursing research to forget that their work is usually conducted in a very different way and setting from that of practicing nurses. Again, this confusion in thinking about nursing is fostered by use of the word *nursing* to refer to both the discipline, which articulates nursing practice, and to the actual practice of nursing care.

Nursing professors must distinguish nursing as a practice from nursing as a discipline. Unlike professors in other practical fields, nursing professors experience both the discipline and the practice. Few political scientists are, in fact, practicing politicians, and professors of education rarely teach in public schools. Professors of nursing, however, because they both practice and study the practice, are in a privileged position to articulate their practice. But for this privilege to be realized, they must succeed in distinguishing the practice of nursing from the discipline of nursing. Nursing practice is experienced as caring for persons who are ill or debilitated or who need assistance to improve or maintain their health. The person cared for is the patient/client and the care given is the practice. The discipline of nursing is experienced as systematic study or research. What is studied is the practice of caring for persons who need assistance related to their health and well being. In short, both the what and the how of the discipline of nursing are very different from that of the practice of nursing.

It seems odd that neither Berit nor Susan, on entering the academy, followed the most obvious, simple, and direct way of articulating nursing, namely, as a caring practice. Indeed it is strange that when nursing preparation, research, and study entered the academy, it looked to the sciences and applied sciences to articulate its essence, rather than articulating nursing as a caring practice—traditionally the source of its identity. Undoubtedly, some nursing scholars were tempted to interpret nursing as a science or as an applied science because nursing, like other practical areas such as business and education, was labelled a science in the academy. However, had these scholars attempted to articulate the essence of nursing as a caring practice, they probably would have found it very difficult to do. At that time, the philosophy of practice was just being rediscovered by Continental philosophers who were treating the human sciences with phenomenological and hermeneutical methods.

In the past, nursing has not been adequately articulated as a caring practice because it had not found its voice. In fact, most of those who have called nursing a practice have had little understanding of what constitutes a practice. Unfortunately, recently some who have called nursing a practice have been narrow traditionalists opposed to change and wedded to the view that nursing is primarily methodology learned by repetition. Phenomenological interpretation, however, has remedied this situation by giving nursing a way of articulating itself as a caring practice that reveals it to be much more sophisticated and intelligible than either the "traditionalists" or the advocates of science could have imagined.

PHENOMENOLOGICAL INTERPRETATION

Phenomenology attempts to disclose the essential meaning of human endeavors. For disclosing the meaning of nursing, the broad, rather than narrow, definition of phenomenology set forth by J. N. Mohanty (1990) is suitable.

> The word 'phenomenology' is often used in a broad, liberal, open-ended sense in which the only constraint on its application is laid down by the imperative of validating one's theoretical-cognitive claims, and of clarifying one's meanings, by the evidence of originary experience. In a narrower, historically grounded sense, one means by 'phenomenology' Husserl's work, and whatever carries that work forward in conformity with its guiding intention. (pp. 7–8)

Like most contemporary phenomenologists, we work from within the Continental tradition rather than from a particular allegiance to Husserl or, for that matter, to any of the other founders of the Continental tradition, such as Heidegger. As such, we will focus on developing an interpretation of nursing from within the Continental tradition while avoiding the complexities and in-fighting that would make that tradition inaccessible to those unacquainted with it. Nonetheless, we will follow what Mohanty contends is true of all phenomenologists: We will seek the meaning of nursing in the lived experience of the practice of nursing and will ask our readers to test our interpretation against their lived experience. Thus, we will not follow traditional philosophy, either by arguing that our interpretation is rationally more adequate than others or by offering a metaphysical or theoretical system as a foundation for nursing. Instead, we will draw out the essential meaning of nursing and test our interpretation of nursing as a caring practice against the lived experience of nursing. In this way we can determine if a phenomenological interpretation of nursing clarifies with greater accuracy and depth than a scientific or technological interpretation.

Paul Ricoeur (1977) offers a broad definition of phenomenology and hermeneutics which is especially appropriate for grasping the meaning of nursing. He defines phenomenology as that philosophy which is concerned with meaning, gives meaning in terms of essence, and discloses essence in terms of a well-chosen example (pp. 145–147). According to Ricoeur, hermeneutics, the theory and practice of interpretation, discloses meanings, especially those that go unrecognized in the normal progress of lived experience (Ricoeur, 1970, pp. 20–36). Since we are working from within the Continental tradition, we will not distinguish between what is disclosed phenomenologically and hermeneutically but will simply use the term phenomenological interpretation to include both. In so doing, we also are replacing the academic term, *hermeneutics*, with its equivalent English term, *interpretation*.

A phenomenological interpretation of nursing seeks to disclose the essential meaning that is found in the lived experience of nurses. In our technological society, however, there is a tendency, when grasping such meaning, to separate meaning from doing. For example, a reviewer of our recent book on nursing and the phenomenology of practice claimed that the thesis of our book is that "nursing is what nurses do" (Chambliss, 1991, p. 72). In treating what nurses do in that way, the reviewer both missed the point of our book and revealed his own bias. In that book, we contended as we do here, that the essence of nursing is disclosed as a way of being with others which is informed by a system of meaning that orders what nurses do in caring for others. Most nurses implicitly grasp the system of meaning which informs their practice. This implicit grasp of meaning takes the form of an unrecognized logic that informs practice. A primary purpose of phenomenological interpretation is to bring to consciousness the unrecognized logic that informs what nurses do. Thus, by phenomenological interpretation, we will bring to consciousness the implicit system of meaning that informs nursing practice.

PHENOMENOLOGICAL INTERPRETATION AND SCIENTIFIC TECHNOLOGY

Since contemporary theories of nursing draw heavily on scientific technology to understand nursing, we will contrast this approach with that of phenomenological interpretation. Science searches for causes that explain certain events, and technology uses these explanations to intervene or control occurrences in desired ways. In scientific explanations, terms have one meaning fixed by scientific theory. Furthermore, science abstracts theory from human experience and uses the theories to impose abstract meaning on things in the world. Again, technology uses these abstract meanings to intervene in natural processes so as to control them in desired ways. Because natural phenomena are not meaningful in and of themselves, science and technology work with such imposed meaning. In contrast, human activities in the world, such as nursing, are meaningful activities, and as such can be understood only in terms of their own meaning rather than through meanings imposed on them. As such, phenomenological interpretation attempts to disclose the human meaning of such practices as nursing rather than imposing meaning on them. Since these meanings are derived from an ongoing practice in the world rather than imposed by abstract theory, they often have hidden implications or double meanings and, therefore, require interpretation to disclose these meanings.

The difference between scientific-technological explanations and phenomenological interpretations in health care are illustrated in the following two examples. The scientific-technological approach to health care attempts to find the cause of an illness, then to define illness as disease on the basis of cause, and finally to discover ways of intervening in the cause, thus bringing about cure. A clear example of this procedure would be that followed with a patient who was psychologically disturbed because of glandular dysfunction. A physician discovered that the patient had had a rare disease, Hashimoto's Thyroiditis, as an adolescent which caused her pituitary gland to malfunction. He gave her chemicals which supplemented the thyroid supply in her body. This, in turn, cured her psychological disturbance. In the foregoing case, the explanation and intervention of scientific technology was appropriate. However, it is inappropriate when used in a case in which the primary difficulty concerns human meaning and relationships. For example, consider the case of a middle-aged nurse who is under great tension because she does not like nursing. Her tension leads to a chemical imbalance which eventuates in what is diagnosed as a psychological disturbance. In this case, unlike the former case, the chemical system of her body is working as it should in response to tension. If her physician gives her chemicals, they function palliatively because they do not treat the reason for her psychological problem. We use the term *reason* because we are not dealing with a cause as in the first case. If the patient's condition is to be really improved, a therapist must help her interpret the meaning of her situation. This requires that the therapist, rather than finding a cause and intervening in it, will help her to understand the reasons for her problem and how to improve her situation.

The therapist may, in exploring the meaning of the patient's illness, discover meanings which are not obvious. For example, therapeutic dialogue reveals that the patient initially became a nurse as a result of pressure from her father, who was a prominent physician. He actually had wanted a son to follow in his footsteps. Instead, he had a daughter who, according to his traditional beliefs, could not be a physician. Therefore, he pressured her into nursing. She now wants to quit nursing but her husband, who has a dominating personality like her father, refuses to allow her to do so. He argues that they need the money her nursing salary contributes to the family finances and contends that it is very unlikely that she could find a job with an equivalent salary. Her problem is greater than a vocational change; it involves learning to take direction of her own life. In this case, interpretation discloses meanings that are not apparent in initially disclosed meanings. This example also involves what Huston Smith (1965, pp. 13-40) contends are the two fundamental meanings of meaning. One concerns the meaning of a word such as *nursing*. What is the meaning of nursing? The other concerns the worth of what we are involved in. What does nursing contribute to the meaning of my life? What does the nurse's dislike of nursing actually mean? Does it mean that she really dislikes nursing or does it mean that she dislikes being dominated by males? Can it be said that she really has experienced being a nurse if she has been one only to please dominant males rather than from a desire to care for patients authentically as do most nurses?

The differences between the scientific-technological and the phenomenological interpretation approaches to the study of health care can be further clarified by contrasting the meanings of illness and disease. Persons experience illness as a disruption in their lives as lived. A stroke is experienced as a failure of the lived body, often as an inability to reach out and grasp things and to move toward things in accustomed ways. In contrast, in medical science a stroke is understood as a cause, usually a thrombus, embolus, or hemorrhage, which impairs blood supply to certain parts of the brain. The cause of the disease is identified by abstract scientific explanation which is often unknown to the patient. When possible, technology is used to intervene in the cause of the disease. Since the patient's knowledge of disease is limited, his or her involvement in such diagnosis and procedures usually consists of giving or denying consent for treatment. In contrast, the patient can and usually does describe the meaning of what is occurring to him or her as illness. Nurses can help interpret the meaning of the experience of the stroke by attempting to reveal its essence and to explore meanings which are not evident to the patient. When the nurse helps the patient understand the meaning of the experience of illness, the nurse often uses phenomenological interpretation without actually realizing it. Many contemporary nursing scholars purposefully use phenomenological interpretation to describe experiences of illness and treatment.

Our use of phenomenological interpretation to describe illness and treatment here is done usually to illuminate the meaning of nursing itself. Nursing concerns meaningful activity and not causal behavior. When one attempts to make sense of nursing, one looks for meanings not for causes. It makes sense to ask what is the meaning of nursing but little sense to ask what is the cause of nursing.

THE TWO TECHNOLOGIES
AND NURSING EDUCATION

Although the meaning of nursing itself cannot be understood causally, the meaning of what nurses do often does rely on causal explanation. For example, a nurse could simply explain to a patient that turning prevented bedsores, or she could explain that the reason for turning is that lying in one position too long restricts the circulation to the tissues and creates decubitus ulcers. The former explanation is an example of traditional craft-technological explanation, the latter case is an example of scientific-technological explanation. Ortega y Gasset (1961) distinguishes between these two types of technology. In craft technology, craftsmen, in making things over a long period of time, gradually improve their techniques. Ancient Greek technology is an excellent example of craft technology. In fact, the Greeks used the word *techné* to designate this type of activity. From the word *techné*, we get the words *technique, technical, technician,* and *technology.* In the West, according to Ortega, craft technology first became scientific technology when the invention of technology became a conscious activity. Then new technique, rather than developing out of a long tradition of craftsmanship, resulted from the deliberate activities of inventors attempting to improve technological efficiency. The final step in the development of scientific technology resulted from applying the theories of science to human problems in order to achieve desired ends. We will refer to the older technology as craft technology and to the more recent development as scientific technology.

Over the past several decades, much of the conflict in nursing education has arisen between those who favor craft technology and those who advocate scientific technology. Craft technologists tend to regard the learning of nursing as acquiring time-tested techniques learned from apprenticeships, especially in hospitals. The scientific technologists believe that nursing can be learned theoretically and later applied to nursing practice. Their approach often is associated with academic schools of nursing. However, the advocates of scientific technology had just gained a firm foothold in the academy when they found themselves threatened by the advocates of the new curriculum. This challenge was bolstered by the use of phenomenological interpretation to reject the positivistic orientation of the advocates of science and technology in nursing.

The technological meaning of nursing education is evident in some of the criticism levied against the new curriculum. Malasanos (1991), a noted critic of the new curriculum, contends that the new curriculum will make nursing unacceptable to the academic community. She believes that in order for nursing to be respectable in the academic community it will have to conform to an academically acceptable model.

That model sets forth learning objectives and the learning experiences that are supposed to assure that students achieve the objectives, and then evaluates the curriculum by how well the objectives have been achieved. Certainly, such a model conforms to a major pattern of organization which often is uncritically accepted in our technological society. But what Malasanos regards as an academic approach is actually a technological approach. It employs a means-ends strategy and uses causal explanation in the weak sense. That is to say, when the weak sense is used in technological explanation, the user often is unaware of its meaning since the effects of the causes are only *probable* rather than *necessary*. In the above case, Malasanos' academic (technological) approach assumes that following a prescribed curriculum will probably cause students to achieve certain objectives. A nursing school curriculum can be assessed using (weak) causal explanations by assuming that if most students understand X and can do Y, it is because of having experienced curriculum Q.

Rather than originating in the academic community, the above technological procedure was developed for making material products. If we want a car to perform in a certain way, we design it and manufacture it to achieve objectives, and then test its performance against our objectives. But can human beings be taught to care for other human beings in this way? Human beings, after all, are not raw materials to be modeled to meet our desires or objectives. Human beings have their own meanings and purposes and respond in very different ways to our efforts to control their behavior. William James, a significant contributor to American psychology and philosophy, actually fostered this diversity of response by challenging students in his classes so as to encourage them to think for themselves (Scudder, 1980). James, also a pluralist, did not believe that his goal of evoking creative individual thought was the only or necessarily the best way to educate. He applauded other professors with teaching styles and objectives that were far different from his own. How can the different styles of teachers that evoke different responses in particular students be included in a fixed curriculum to be evaluated by fixed objectives? Similarly, how could a technological approach to nursing curriculum encourage nurses to creatively develop their own way of caring for patients in ways appropriate to particular patients in different situations? A procedure which is appropriate for making products seems inappropriate for teaching human begins to care for other human beings. Caring for other human beings, after all, concerns a way of relating to them, not a means of forming them into products.

The technological way of thinking about and organizing nursing education is being challenged in our so-called postmodern era. A new generation of nursing scholars is challenging the technological model of Ralph Tyler that has dominated interpretations of nursing education for the past 35 years (Bevis & Watson, 1989, p. 2). What is needed to support their efforts is not only defense of the new curriculum but also philosophical critique of the technological articulation of nursing and development of an alternate interpretation of nursing as a caring practice that is academically defensible—thus, our critique and alternate, phenomenological interpretation of nursing as practiced. Our primary purpose, however, is not specifically to support the new curriculum but to improve the quality of nursing care through better understanding of its meaning.

A phenomenological interpretation of nursing is not primarily academic, in the sense that it aims at articulating the meaning of nursing as an end in itself. Although such treatment might be fascinating to a philosopher of the human sciences, such as Scudder, our primary purpose is to help nurses more fully understand the meaning of nursing so that they can better care for their patients/clients and improve nursing practice itself. Stephen Strasser (1985) calls this kind of study practical human science to distinguish it from theoretical human science, which is aimed primarily at understanding something for its own sake. All human science differs from natural science in that human science studies human artifacts and activities which, unlike natural phenomena, have meaning built into them by human beings. The primary purpose of human science is to articulate and interpret that human meaning. This overall purpose is achieved in ways which distinguish the theoretical human sciences from the practical human sciences. According to Strasser, the theoretical human sciences are primarily aimed at "scientific description of the social, cultural, historical world or some of its sections" (pp. 73–76). In contrast, the practical human sciences "have as their aim the articulation and improvement of . . . practices" (pp. 73–76). Improving practice involves developing better practice to be handed on to future generations as well as fostering better practice by individual practitioners in given situations. This work attempts to help practicing nurses and nursing scholars articulate and improve nursing practice through phenomenological interpretation of their important human endeavors.

2

The Discipline of Nursing

Much of the confusion concerning nursing comes from the fact that the term *nursing* is used to signify both the practice of nursing care and the discipline of nursing through which that care is studied. Separating the practice of nursing from the discipline of nursing is difficult because the discipline of nursing actually studies the practice of nursing care. In addition, both have the goal of fostering excellent practice. Since the discipline of nursing is constituted by the study of nursing care, any discussion of the discipline will necessarily involve describing the practice of nursing. Thus, while focused on the discipline of nursing, this chapter also contains considerable treatment of the practice of nursing. In fact, this is so much the case that much of the treatment of what constitutes the practice of nursing is actually in this chapter rather than in the following chapter on the practice of nursing.

Nursing as a practice and nursing as a discipline can be distinguished from each other because nursing care is given very differently from the way in which that care is studied. For example, in this book we are studying the practice of nursing by engaging in phenomenological interpretation to disclose the meaning of nursing as practiced. Nursing practice, however, is not constituted by phenomenological interpretation but by a system of meaning that informs nursing activity that has developed over time.

In this chapter, we will examine the two primary ways of engaging in a phenomenological interpretation of nursing. The first discloses the meaning of nursing care by the direct study of that care. The second interprets the meaning of nursing in light of philosophical treatments of the meaning of human existence.

EXCELLENCE IN NURSING PRACTICE: BENNER

Benner (1984) engaged in phenomenological interpretation of direct nursing care to make an extensive study of nursing practice. From this study she was able to determine the competencies required for giving excellent nursing care. Her primary method, interpreting individual and small group interviews and making interpretive observations of practicing nurses, enabled her to identify 31 competencies of nursing practice which she then grouped under seven domains:

> the helping function, the teaching-coaching function, the diag-
> nostic-monitoring function, effective management of rapidly
> changing situations, administering and monitoring therapeu-
> tic intervention and regimens, monitoring and ensuring the
> quality of health care practices, and organizational and work-
> role competencies. (p. 46)

We will illustrate Benner's (1984) articulation of nursing by discussing one exemplar from her book. This example illustrates the domain of the helping role which includes the following eight competencies:

> The healing relationship: Creating a climate for and establish-
> ing a commitment to healing.
>
> Providing comfort measures and preserving personhood in the
> face of pain and extreme breakdown.
>
> Presencing: Being with a patient.
>
> Maximizing the patient's participation and control in his or
> her own recovery.
>
> Interpreting kinds of pain and selecting appropriate strategies
> for pain management and control.
>
> Providing comfort and communication through touch.
>
> Providing emotional and informational support to patient's
> families.

Guiding a patient through emotional and developmental change: Providing new options, closing off old ones: Channeling, teaching, meditation. (p. 50)

We chose the competency of maximizing the patient's participation and control in his or her own recovery to illustrate how Benner discloses the essence of nursing practice with an appropriate example. In this exemplar of nursing excellence, a nurse cared for a concert pianist who had suffered a mild stroke and was depressed over the weakness in her right hand.

I just sat down and listened and talked to her. I did not say that I wanted her to go to physical therapy, but that was my intention. I said to her that she was showing some progress. "Think about two days ago; today you can move your fingers a little bit more. You have made progress because of the exercise. If you keep doing these exercises, I expect that you will be able to have more use of your hands." I encouraged her—pointing out the positive things because she was only zeroing in on the negative things and looking at how much she didn't have. I reminded her that when she first came in that her arm was weak and that she needed a lot of help to eat. Now she is able to hold a cup by herself. Now she is able to move her fingers and raise her arm; she could even raise it over her head. I said, "Look, you couldn't do that yesterday and you are able to do that today." I just went through all the things that I could see that I hadn't seen the day before. After our talk she went to physical therapy. (pp. 59–60)

In the above case excellent care is given in a routine, rather than exceptional, situation. At some point in their daily care, most nurses have encouraged a patient to engage in physical therapy or some other treatment. The nurse's excellence here is evident in the manner she relates to the patient: She does not violate the patient's integrity by engaging in manipulative tactics. Through straightforward but creative dialogue, the nurse helps the patient to see that she needs to engage in therapy and gently encourages her to do so.

Benner begins not with theories but with nursing practice. Therefore, rather than using some theoretical commitment to decide what constitutes excellent nursing, she begins with those exemplars that nurses themselves consider excellent practice. Then Benner proceeds to disclose what constitutes excellent practice. Through narrative interview and dialogue, she and her colleagues are able to articulate the essence of excellent practice. But her articulation is not done with fundamental concepts, followed by a set of adjectives defining those concepts. Instead, she presents the meaning of such competencies as maximizing the patient's participation and control in his or her own recovery through an example which is interpreted. For instance, Benner (1984) provides the following interpretation of the above case:

> The nurse helps the patient regain a sense of control and active participation in recovery. Many patients feel alienated from their recovery and treatment; frequently it is the nurse who assists the patient in regaining a sense of participation and control. (p. 61)

Benner's treatment of competencies describes how the good at which nursing aims is accomplished, both for the patient and the nurses themselves. For instance, in the above example of nursing excellence, the nurse, by engaging in dialogue in an encouraging way, helps a patient to recognize and to choose the therapy that will restore mobility to her arm and hand, thus making it possible for her to play the piano again. The nurse does this by helping the patient to recognize how far she has progressed but also that further therapy is needed. Unlike some nursing care, however, that tends to foster patient helplessness, this nurse's care fosters patient independence in at least two ways. First, she fosters hope by helping the patient see what she has already accomplished, and suggesting the possibility of future accomplishment. Second, she encourages the patient to make her own decision. Of course, one could object that she has set the context of decision making in such a way as to help ensure that the patient will decide for therapy. However, her expert understanding of health care indicates to her that therapy is needed if the patient is to recover the use of her arm. Choices made by patients during nursing care are not ends in themselves, as those who overstress autonomy often imply, but instead involve making choices that determine whether or not the good at which nursing practice aims is accomplished. In the above case as presented, the need for therapy seems obvious and clear, and there are no conflicting alternatives. Cases presented in nursing etl. often contain conflicting alternatives. For example, in the above conflict might have been evident if the therapy was very expensiv ...d the patient very poor with a large family in financial difficulty due to the cost of the patient's hospitalization. But the fact that conflicting interests often are used in nursing classes to highlight various aspects of nursing care should not obscure the fact that decisions in nursing care often do not involve such conflicts. Many times they are uncomplicated, as in the above case—a concert pianist has had a stroke and needs to recover the use of her arm. What she needs, rather than a complicated process for decision making, is the courage to undertake the extensive therapy that is necessary for her to regain the use of her arm and hand. By encouraging the patient to engage in therapy, the nurse is helping the patient develop the courage and the determination needed for recovery. Thus, the patient will gain independence, not only by recovering greater use of her arm, but by the way she decides for and engages in therapy through empowering dialogue with her nurse.

Benner's study of nursing as practiced demonstrates the integral relationship which should exist between the practice of nursing and the discipline of nursing. We say "should exist" because this integral relationship has been torn apart by the tendency of nursing scholars to study nursing with theories and methods drawn from disciplines other than nursing. Benner's study is, at once, a study of nursing practice and a demonstration of how nursing practice can be studied in ways appropriate to the practice. The meaning of nursing excellence is given through exemplars that show nursing competencies as instantiations of excellence. These instantiations of excellence are given through narrative descriptions which convey the meaning of excellence rather than through concepts qualified so as to delineate what counts as excellence. The meaning of these exemplars is further made evident by interpretation. Such interpretation makes it possible to go beyond the obvious meaning of the example to recognition of the process involved in nursing excellence: in the foregoing example, an empowering dialogue that encouraged the patient to undergo the extensive therapy necessary to restore her former abilities. In summary, Benner uses phenomenological interpretation to disclose excellences manifested in nursing practice through well-chosen examples and interprets those examples to make evident less obvious meanings.

THE IN-BETWEEN STANCE IN NURSING:
BISHOP AND SCUDDER

A phenomenological interpretation of nursing, specifically as a practice, was given in our most recent book (Bishop & Scudder, 1990). The central thesis of that book—nursing is a practice with an inherent moral sense—was developed by articulating nursing in light of the philosophy of practice. While an abbreviated treatment of that thesis will be developed in the following chapter, more inquisitive readers are referred to the 1990 volume for a more comprehensive discussion of the subject. Nonetheless, the abbreviated treatment given here will serve as an example of how the discipline of nursing can be enhanced by articulating nursing in light of philosophical interpretation. Specifically, we will treat a controversial thesis of our previous book, namely, the in-between stance of the nurse. We will not treat this stance fully but only as an illustration of how to articulate nursing practice in a way that contributes to the discipline of nursing. After a brief examination of why the in-between stance is necessary in nursing practice, we will clarify the meaning of the in-between stance by interpreting an example of nursing excellence.

In our 1990 volume, we contended that Benner's articulation of nursing excellence establishes an area of legitimate authority particular to nursing that is primarily under the control of nurses. In addition, we contended that nursing is constituted by a distinctive in-between stance. Nurses must work in-between the physician, patient, and agency bureaucrats because nursing practice itself often is constituted by bringing together medical contributions, regulative controls and permissions, and the personal aspirations of patients into systematic and personal daily care.

It was Tristram Engelhardt (1985) who originally viewed the in-between stance of the nurse in a negative light, regarding it as a situation in which nurses were "caught." Timothy Sheard's (1980) phenomenological description of the different work worlds of the physician and nurse amplifies the negative aspect of the in-between. When describing various aspects of the in-between stance, Sheard contended that "the physician 'owns his time' and usually a portion of the nurse's time. He alots the nurse's time by giving orders which require the use of the nurse's time. The nurse's time is also allotted by a hospital schedule with definite and routine requirements to be done according to the clock" (in Bishop & Scudder, 1990, p. 18). Although Sheard's assessment of the nurse's work world is negative when contrasted with that of the physician, it can be put in a much more positive light when placed in a different context. For example, since nurses want to foster the well being of patients, they faithfully execute the sound medical regimens prescribed by physicians. Since nurses require an ordered work place, protection of their rights and privileges, and access to needed equipment and space, they support and to some degree administer agency policy. Finally, since nurses are usually much more closely related to patients than anyone else, they are in a position to know what patients desire and therefore to become advocates for the patient. Stated positively, by working in-between, nurses foster the patient's well being in a uniquely direct way by bringing all the foregoing aspects of health care together into systematic day-to-day care.

Not only does giving daily nursing care require the nurse to work in-between, but, as we have argued extensively elsewhere (Bishop & Scudder, 1987, 1990), the in-between position is a privileged one for making the team decisions required in health care ethics. Making moral decisions in health care requires consideration of what is medically correct, what is institutionally permissible, and what is desired by the patient. Therefore, the person who works in-between is uniquely situated for bringing these perspectives together. However, this process of bringing together these different aspects of health care, including the nurse's own special area of legitimate authority, places the nurse in a very difficult position. It is for this reason that Engelhardt (1985) described the in-between position as one in which nurse's are "caught." Although it is true that the in-between position fosters difficulties for the nurse, it also places nurses in a position uniquely suited to fostering the patient's well being.

Clearly, then, the in-between stance is essential in nursing not because nurses historically have been required to work in this way. The in-between stance is necessary because it is required to give needed daily care. For this reason one could not be a nurse, especially in the hospital, without being able to work in-between. The foregoing statement does not mean, of course, that nurses always work in-between, even in hospitals. Nurses have their own area of legitimate authority which Benner (1984, 1989), to our way of thinking, has articulated with much precision. For example, in the case of the nurse encouraging the stroke patient to undergo physical therapy, the nurse was working within the legitimate authority of nursing. She is in no way in-between the patient, the physician or the hospital bureaucrat. In fact, nurses frequently work within their own area of legitimate authority and need only to cooperate reasonably with other health care workers involved. But nurses also often must work in-between. In actual practice, these two aspects of nursing often are so interrelated that nurses move from one to the other without being overtly aware that they are doing so.

The meaning of the in-between can be made more evident by phenomenological interpretation of the following example.

> A physician was in a quandary concerning whether to aspirate the lungs of a patient who was in an advanced stage of metastatic cancer. The patient suffered from hallucinations, and he often experienced severe pain. In addition, due to heavy smoking, the alveoli no longer functioned adequately. The physician believed that the right medical decision was to let the patient die. He did not discuss this with the patient; in fact, he rarely discussed treatment with anyone including nurses. He was a very technically competent surgeon who believed that he alone should determine the medically correct form of treatment. The nurse knew that the patient was weary of his struggle, felt hopeless and was ready to die. But she also knew that for some reason the patient had struggled to remain alive more valiantly than most other patients for whom she had cared. When she complimented him on his remarkable courage, he responded that he was not remarkably courageous at all. He merely wished to remain alive to celebrate Christmas with his family. The patient had a large family with strong attachments to their father and to each other. The family had a tradition of celebrating Christmas together, and Christmas was a few weeks away. In spite of the fact that the nurse knew that this physician did not receive suggestions concerning treatment from nurses "graciously," she shared her knowledge of the patient's wishes with the physician, and he aspirated the lungs. When the patient's loquacious family arrived to celebrate Christmas, there was much confusion and noise in the Oncology Unit. Complaints were made by other patients, some of whom were also near the end of their lives

and felt they should have peace and quiet during that time and, of course, their wishes were supported by hospital policy. The nurse, knowing of another patient unit where the census was very low due to Christmas, arranged for the patient to be transferred to an isolated room on that unit where other patients would not be disturbed. She even allowed his two-year-old great granddaughter to be "smuggled" into the hospital, which at the time was against hospital policy. (Bishop & Scudder, 1990, pp. 139–140)

In the above example, it is clear that the nurse works in-between. She not only effectively carries out legitimate orders of the physician but makes a suggestion to the physician when the well being of the patient calls for it. Her concern for the patient is evident in her willingness to make a suggestion concerning medical treatment to a physician who did not readily accept such suggestions, especially from nurses. Her knowledge of the hospital system and her ability to work within it make it possible for her to make the arrangements necessary for the patient to enjoy Christmas with his family. But she does this in a way that considers the well being of other patients and in no way threatens hospital order. She is able to do this because she has grasped the purpose for and spirit of hospital order rather than making it an end in itself. She is so attuned to the patient that she is able to draw out his wishes without in any way imposing on him. Her in-between situation includes being available to the family including the great grandchild. In caring for her patient, she becomes an existential advocate of the patient to the physician and to the hospital administration in a way that helps the patient authentically live the end of his life as he wishes to live it (see p. 25 for Gadow's interpretation of existential advocacy).

NARRATIVE STUDY AND THE DISCIPLINE OF NURSING

In discussing how the discipline of nursing can be developed in ways that do not reduce or distort the practice of nursing, we and Benner have employed phenomenological interpretation to articulate nursing practice. In describing these studies, we have introduced narrative study by interpreting narrative descriptions of excellence and of the in-between stance so common to nurses working in hospitals. We will expand this treatment of narrative study as a means of disclosing the practice of nursing by showing how we have used the interpretation of narratives to discern how nurses experience the practice of nursing.

The use of narratives to interpret health care is sometimes received with skepticism by health care professionals. Many health care professionals are suspicious of personal narrative accounts which they often dismiss as mere anecdotes. For example, Norman Cousins (1989) was warned to avoid the use of anecdotes when he joined the faculty of the medical school at UCLA. He soon learned that physicians "are taught to shun conclusions based on single experiences and to look for evidence based on a substantial number of cases" (p. 12). In contrast, he observed that "writers seek out anecdotes as a way of making larger statements" and that in the "writer's world, statistics obscure souls. Whole lives get gobbled up by whole numbers" (p. 12). He learned that for medical researchers truth will be discovered "in a laboratory setting, will be demonstrated, will lend itself to quantification, and will be tested and cross-tested" (p. 13). These objectifying tendencies of contemporary medicine were put in proper perspective by a friend who read Cousins with one of the present authors. This friend had already lived with cancer for two years more than had been predicted by medical prognosis, but now he was faced with symptoms which indicated that his remission had ended. On reading the above passage of Cousins, he retorted, "What physicians called a single instance, I call my life, and what they call a mere anecdote, I call the story of my life."

Medicine, and to a lesser degree nursing, has favored the statistical, scientific approach to knowledge. This approach often works well in categorizing disease by diagnosis and prescribing treatments that have been scientifically shown to be effective. The practices of nursing and medicine, however, are not natural objects, they are human creations. Even so, they often have been studied from a perspective which Husserl (1965) would call the "natural attitude" and Heidegger (1962) would call "objective thinking." These practices have been treated as "things" to be put in a more comprehensive category of like things and distinguished from other similar things. This thing-categorical way of thinking has served the natural sciences well, at least until the mid-twentieth century. But it is difficult, if not impossible, to deal with many aspects of health care adequately when they are conceived of as things to be grasped categorically and studied empirically in the narrow sense.

One aspect of nursing practice that cannot be known scientifically, and especially not statistically, is how nurses experience their practice. Interpreting narratives, however, can disclose significant aspects of the meaning of such experiences. Narratives, according to Donald Polkinghorne (1988), are "the primary form through which humans construct the dimensions of their life's meaningfulness and understand it as significant" (p. 155). In interpreting narratives, one should be aware that "narrative meaning consists of more than the events alone; it consists also of the significance these events have for the narrator in relation to a particular theme" (p. 160). In discovering this significance, the interpreter must reveal not only the meaning of the events of which the narrator is conscious but also those of which he or she may not be aware. Narrative research not only discloses personal meaning but also the "interpretive schemes a people or community uses to establish the significance of past events and to anticipate the consequences of possible future actions" (p. 162). Nursing is the community we have explored, focusing on the experience of fulfillment in nursing practice.

We used narrative interpretation in our study of fulfillment not so much from an interest in demonstrating the efficacy of human science methodology for interpreting nursing but from a desire to know aspects of health care practice which cannot be known using objectifying methodology. We wanted to know what practicing nurses experienced as the essential meaning of being a nurse. From previous experience with nurses, we knew that the stress on objective methodology in their professional education would incline them toward categorical reduction or behavioral description. In the case of categorical reduction, they would describe only those aspects of their practice that conformed to what they had been taught constituted good practice. In the case of behavioral description, they would merely list those activities in which they were typically engaged in their practice. Therefore, we asked for narrative descriptions of their most fulfilling experience in nursing practice. These narratives were primarily written. Follow-up interviews were used to clarify meanings and to test our interpretation of the narratives. Through interpreting these narratives, we drew some surprising conclusions which previous studies of nursing missed because they were wedded to objective methodology.

FULFILLMENT IN NURSING

By using narratives to study nursing, we attempted to discover what practicing nurses experienced as the meaning of being a nurse. We asked them to focus on nursing as practiced by requiring their description in narrative form of the experience in which they felt most fulfilled as a nurse. From the professional literature in nursing, we assumed that most nurses would describe experiences in which they demonstrated unusual professional or technical competency. We did expect to find, however, that more nurses would describe situations in which fulfillment came from satisfying the moral or personal sense of nursing than most professional literature implied. The overwhelming affirmation by our respondents of the moral and personal as the most fulfilling aspect of nursing greatly surprised us. Of the 40 practicing nurses in two community hospitals and a university medical center who participated in the study, all of the nurses' most fulfilling experiences were dominantly moral or personal except for one. Even that nurse had difficulty deciding whether she was most fulfilled by satisfying the moral and personal sense of nursing or by executing technical skills expertly.

From the 40 practicing nurses in our study, we have chosen the following description to exemplify our general finding that nurses are most fulfilled when the moral sense of nursing is achieved in a personal relationship.

> *Two years ago I had the opportunity to deliver total patient care to a 25-year-old girl with end stage congestive cardiomyopathy. She was in congestive heart failure with many ventricular life threatening arrhythmias. She was well aware of the fact that she was going to die and admitted her fright to me and also asked me point blank if she was going to die. We were able to discuss such problems as how could this be explained to her 7-year-old daughter? Who would care for her 7-year-old daughter and her own 16-year-old retarded sister? I also discussed with her family some of the fears she acknowledged and encouraged them to discuss these things with her. Her main request of me was that I sit by her during the night and simply hold her hand. In addition to ministering to these needs, I also*

monitored her vital signs, changes in physical assessment, ti-
trating various vasopressors and vasodilators to maintain opti-
mum cardiac output. I overrode our strict visiting policies to
allow her husband and daughter to sit at her bedside as they
wished with the understanding that they would promptly leave
if asked to do so by any of us. This patient remained in my unit
for 4–5 weeks in critical condition before dying and though we
all felt the hurt of losing her, we also felt the joy obtained by
providing emotional and physical support along with patient
teaching to both patient and family and helped both patient
and family to accept and begin to deal with her inevitable
death. (Scudder & Bishop, 1990, pp. 146–147)

In the above narrative it is evident that the dominant reason for the
nurse's fulfillment came from her moral sense of having fostered the
patient's well being in an extremely trying situation and from her
intense personal relationship with the patient. However, it is significant to note that although the primary fulfillment from her nursing
care is personal and moral, her care incorporates a highly technical
aspect of nursing practice. Although a physician is not mentioned, the
nature of the technical aspect of her care surely required her to work
in-between the physician and the patient. She obviously works in-
between the patient and the hospital and the patient and her family.
Not only is she an excellent exemplar of working in-between, she also
is an excellent exemplar of what Gadow calls an "existential advocate."
Her advocacy extends beyond that usually related to everyday nursing
care to that aspect of advocacy which is decidedly existential, namely,
facing one's own death.

EXISTENTIAL ADVOCACY: GADOW

In this chapter we have employed philosophical methodology, specifically phenomenological interpretation, to disclose the meaning of
nursing. If such disclosure is understood to be *the* only possible meaning of nursing, it can limit development of future nursing practice and
isolate it from other human ventures. For this reason nursing needs to
be interpreted in light of philosophical, and other, interpretations of

the meaning of human existence that suggest the future possible development of nursing. For example, Sally Gadow (1980) suggests a possible enhancement of nursing by interpreting nursing as existential advocacy. She explores the meaning of nursing in light of the contention of existential phenomenology that the primary meaning of being human is to be self-directing. Gadow shows how nursing can foster authentic human being in persons facing illness, treatment, and possible death.

Enlightening practice by philosophical interpretation, however, is not confined to existential phenomenology. Israel Scheffler (1966), an analytic philosopher, has enlightened educational practice by drawing on classical philosophers. He states, "I make no pretense to historical accuracy. My main purpose is . . . to see what, if anything, each [philosophy] has to offer us in our own quest for a satisfactory conception of teaching" (p. 174). Like Scheffler, in this book we will focus our interpretation on the meaning of nursing itself and will treat the philosophies of practice, caring, and personal relationships in ways that will enlighten our understanding of nursing.

Interpreting practice in light of philosophical interpretations of the meaning of human existence is different from the foundational approach to philosophy, common to nursing and education. Those who follow the foundation approach assume that nursing must be founded on some system of philosophy in order to be a valid enterprise. This system is then used to prescribe what constitutes good nursing. In contrast, interpreting practice in light of philosophy assumes that practices such as nursing have made and continue to make significant contributions to human life. However, understanding that contribution requires an interpretation of nursing as a human endeavor. Interpretations of nursing in light of specific philosophies explore the present or possible contributions of nursing to fostering the full humanity of those needing health care.

Gadow's interpretation of nursing, generated by existential phenomenology, elaborates a major theme of that philosophy itself: "freedom of self-determination is the most fundamental and valuable human right" (p. 84). This, of course, means that nurses should assist patients to become self-determining in ways that express "the full and unique complexity of their values" (p. 97). This requires nurses to relate to patients as whole persons by bringing together the personal and professional (p. 97) and the lived body and the body object (pp. 93–96). Gadow succinctly summarizes existential advocacy as "participating with the patient in determining the personal meaning which the experience of illness, suffering, or dying is to have for that individual" (p. 97).

The strength of Gadow's contention lies in its call for nurses to assist patients to become self-determining whole human beings. What makes nurses likely candidates for existential advocacy is that they often come to know patients well at a time when they are very vulnerable and are seeking help, counsel, and direction. In such situations nurses are those who are there and usually available.

Although Gadow contends that existential advocacy is different from traditional nursing, it actually is not if nursing is interpreted as Benner and we articulate it. For example, the nurse who encouraged the pianist with the stroke to engage in therapy is helping her to become what she wants to be. In so doing, this nurse is an exemplar of one type of existential advocacy. All nurses should help patients overcome limitations, fears, doubts, and anxieties due to their illness and treatment which prevent them from regaining the lost powers and abilities necessary for becoming what they want to be. An exemplar of another type of advocacy necessary for nurses was the nurse who helped the dying patient celebrate Christmas as he wished by becoming his advocate to the physician and in the hospital. Obviously, a nurse makes an excellent choice as existential advocate because she is situated in-between the physician, patient, and hospital bureaucracy. Both of the foregoing are exemplars of existential advocacy in traditional nursing practice at its best, the first as articulated by Benner and the second as we articulated it. Thus, existential advocacy is not so much a redirection of traditional nursing as it is a possibility for its further realization.

CONCLUSION

In this chapter, we have shown how phenomenological interpretation can contribute to developing the discipline of nursing. We have explored two ways of engaging in such phenomenological interpretation. We have used Gadow's interpretation of nursing as existential advocacy as an example of how nursing can be interpreted philosophically as a significant human venture. Because we will illustrate this further in the following chapters by interpreting nursing in light of philosophies of practice and caring, we will focus this conclusion on the other approach discussed: phenomenological interpretations of narrative descriptions of practice. Narrative descriptions are important in the study of nursing because they direct nurses to their lived experience which is often obscured by professional education and literature that inclines nurses to think and speak objectively. When nurses describe their practice narratively, they treat it fundamentally as a moral activity focused on personal relationships with patients. In contrast, much of professional literature implies that nursing is a scientific or technological undertaking. Our studies and Benner's show that narrative descriptions direct practitioners to their lived experience, and interpretation of these narratives discloses dimensions of practice missed by the objective methodologies that categorize and quantify practices.

At the beginning of the chapter, we contended that phenomenological interpretation of the discipline of nursing discloses the practice of nursing care. Benner's study has disclosed an area of legitimate authority in nursing practice that nurses control. She describes this area in terms of competencies that foster excellent nursing. Our study has shown that nursing also is constituted by an in-between stance that is necessary for giving daily care and that is a privileged position from which to foster the team decisions required in health care ethics. Our narrative study of fulfillment in nursing indicates that practicing nurses experience nursing primarily as a moral and personal human endeavor. Gadow's study, by advocating that nurses become existential advocates, suggests a possible way of improving nursing practice. These phenomenological interpretations of nursing indicate that nursing is a caring practice. Further development of this meaning of nursing requires that nursing be interpreted in light of philosophies of practice and of caring.

3

Nursing as Practice

Through its long history, nursing has tended to identify itself as a caring practice. Unfortunately, the meaning of caring practice has only recently begun to be articulated by nursing scholars. Strangely, this articulation has come after and partly in response to the attempt of nursing scholars to define nursing as a science or an applied science. As we have pointed out in previous chapters, the definition of nursing as a science or an applied science is related to nursing education's move to the academy. The academy has no place for the study of practices. Traditionally, universities were divided into the arts and sciences. Recently, the applied sciences and social sciences have been added. It would make sense for a university to have a division of the practical human sciences, but, in fact, no such division exists, so practices such as nursing are usually included within the sciences or applied sciences. However, the practice of nursing itself certainly could not be a science. Sciences aim at knowing the truth as an end in itself, whereas practices attempt to bring about good in the world: in the case of nursing the promotion and maintenance of good health. Nursing could be called an applied science on the other hand; nurses do apply science to practical areas in order to bring about good health. Treating nursing as an applied science is at least a possible alternative to treating it as a practice. Since nursing traditionally has been considered a practice, any change of definition to applied science requires that the burden of proof be on those advocating that change. Such proof should require a consideration of the meaning of applied science and its implications for nursing. However, when the meaning of applied science or technology is considered, difficulties arise in choosing this alternative. After discussing these difficulties we will consider the meaning of practice, drawing on two philosophers of practice, Hans George Gadamer (1981) and Alisdair MacIntyre (1984). The consideration of the meaning of technology and of practice should make it evident that the reinterpretation of nursing from a practice to a technology is unwarranted.

Following the phenomenological interpretation approach, we will begin to explore the meaning of technology by example. Two radar technicians in the U.S. Army Air Force during World War II were arguing about the nature of technical competence. One of the technicians was excellent in the theoretical side of technology but inept in the mechanical side. The other was very adept in the mechanical side but very poor in the theoretical side. As the argument proceeded, the mechanically competent technician attempted to make his case by asking the theorist, "What will you would do when they send you to the South Pacific and there is no one there to help you solder?" To which the theorist responded, "What will you do when you are in the South Pacific and there is no one there to tell you how this thing works?" This technician clearly recognized that being a competent technician requires, above all, proficiency in theoretical explanation. Those who fail to grasp this will consider practice more important than theory, but by practice they mean methodology or technique. Thus, although the primary technological struggle is usually stated as being between theory and practice, it is actually between theory and methodology. In nursing, this argument is between those who advocate scientific technology and those who favor craft technology. Benner (1984) does, in fact, contend that both forms of technology are necessary in nursing. But she conclusively shows that expert nursing cannot be constituted as either craft or scientific technology. Expert nursing requires that nurses use both technologies creatively within the context of meaning of a caring practice. Such a practice, as Benner convincingly shows, can only be learned clinically.

In contrast to being learned clinically, scientific technology is learned primarily by studying theory and how that theory is applied to achieve certain desired outcomes. One becomes a technician by learning theory and its application rather than through clinical experience. The significance of this can be made evident by considering the possibility of Scudder becoming a nurse. Obviously, after years of studying the philosophy and the theory of nursing, he is certainly more versed in that area than most practicing nurses. In fact, he has earned many CEU credits as a result of attending nursing conferences at which he read papers concerned with the theoretical side of nursing. If nursing were a scientific technology, he could become a nurse by enrolling in a program that would show him how to apply his theoretical understanding to practical situations. The fact that it would be ludicrous to initiate novices into nursing in this way is a strong indication that nursing is not a scientific technology. Nursing education's heavy reliance on clinical experience is a strong indication that it is, in fact, a practice.

Another strong indication that nursing is not a technology is that personal factors are very important in nursing excellence, whereas, personal qualities are insignificant in technology. To be a good technician, one needs only the requisite theoretical understanding and the ability to apply that understanding to specific projects. A technician may be pleasant or personable on or off the job but this has little to do with technological competence. In contrast, personal qualities are very important in nursing. Nurses must be able to relate to others personally, possess a sensitive therapeutic touch, and be sensitive to the desires and feelings of other people. This was evident in a study of personality traits valued by nurses in which nurturance, sentience, and understanding were ranked both by practicing nurses and students as the dominant personality traits required in nursing (Bradham, Dalme, & Thompson, 1990, 231-232). In nursing, personality factors are not add-on aspects desirable for nurses to possess but are necessary for excellent nursing. For example, many nursing educators have had the unpleasant task of counseling out of nursing who were excellent academic students who could well perform the skills of nursing but whose personality made it very unlikely that they would ever be a successful nurse.

Since nursing is learned primarily through clinical experience rather than by learning and applying theory and it stresses unique personal relationships rather than uniform impersonal processes, nursing is a poor candidate for becoming an applied science. Why, then, should nursing scholars attempt to restructure nursing as an applied science? It is tempting here to say that the primary reason for this designation (nursing is an applied science) is the fact that nursing usually has been placed with the theoretical and applied sciences in the academy. The larger issue, at stake, of course, is why nursing and other practices have been labelled as sciences rather than practices in the academy? Gadamer (1981) suggests this reason: In the Western world "the hour of technology has arrived by way of science" (p. 70). Gadamer also contends that the rise of technology has led to the "degeneration of practice into technique" (p. 69). What Gadamer and others are trying to do is to help the Western world recover its lost sense of practice.

THE MEANING OF PRACTICE: GADAMER AND MACINTYRE

Gadamer (1981) recounts how the sense of practice has been lost in the West by returning to the Greek origins of both practice and technology. The philosophy of practice had been a primary concern of the Greeks, especially Aristotle. Aristotle contended that good practice came about as a result of practical wisdom. Practical wisdom was concerned with bringing about the good in social, political, and personal affairs. With practical wisdom he contrasted theoretical wisdom which was concerned with knowing the rational order (logos) on which the world was founded. Theoretical wisdom provided the model out of which modern science eventually developed. When that knowledge was later applied to changing the world, it received the name *technology*, which came from combining two Greek words, *logos* and *techné*. Logos signified the rational order of the universe which theoretical wisdom was supposed to disclose, and techné designated the know-how that came from applying theoretical knowledge to the world. This conception of applied theory (technology) has risen to a place of prominence in the Western world never imagined by the Greeks. The Greeks associated techné with the making of things rather than with human relations and communal institutions. Science and technology gained new prominence in the West when they were applied to human affairs through the social sciences in the latter part of the nineteenth century.

Initially, the social sciences tended to be modelled after the natural sciences. Those who followed this tendency to its logical conclusion transformed the social sciences into the behavioral sciences. The tendency to reduce the social sciences to behavioral sciences has been challenged by the rise of the human sciences. The human sciences, in contrast to the behavioral sciences, sought to develop a discipline appropriate to the study of man and human affairs. The human sciences, especially as developed in contemporary Continental thought, revived the philosophy of practice begun by the Greeks. Rather than focusing on knowledge and its use, practice articulates how the particular good inherent in the practice is accomplished in the world. Thus, it is very different from technology which applies scientific knowledge to the world in order to change it. As we will attempt to make clear, nursing is primarily concerned with bringing about its inherent good in the world. The primary way in which nursing brings about that good is not by applying science but by the practice of caring.

The manner by which Gadamer distinguishes practice from technology is helpful in disclosing why nursing is a practice rather than a technology. Technology concerns techniques derived from scientific knowledge. Its aim is to control or intervene in some aspect of the world. This control or intervention can be, and often is, used to bring about something that is considered as good. However, technology itself is neutral; it can as easily be used to foster that which is considered as undesirable or evil as good. In contrast, the goal of a practice is to bring about a particular good in the world in ways which are integrally related to the good sought. Thus, a practice is founded on the good it is designed to achieve and makes no sense apart from it.

Health care professionals often become aware of the moral sense of their practice when it is replaced or challenged by goals other than the good that health care is designed to achieve. For example, when the free enterprise logic of the bottom line becomes the dominant sense of medicine, the patient does not know whether or not to trust his or her physician. Is the physician suggesting an expensive operation because of a desire to heal the patient or to purchase a new swimming pool? Nurses also are subject to rejecting the sense of their practice by pursuing alien goals. For example, a nurse might continually give patients pain medication just to keep them sedated so that the nurse can complete administrative forms unrelated to nursing duties. While completing such forms might ingratiate the nurse with the executive director of the hospital, by doing so, the nurse would not be following the moral sense of nursing practice, but the logic of bureaucracy which calls for advancement by pleasing superiors and following institutional rules. When a nurse, including a nursing administrator, becomes more concerned with bureaucratic goals and procedures than with fostering the well being of patients, he or she ceases being a nurse and becomes a bureaucrat.

A practice not only has a dominant moral sense that provides its meaning, according to Gadamer (1981), but it also provides a sense of identity to practitioners. This sense of identity comes from making choices concerning how the inherent good is to be achieved. In contrast, a technological system takes away choices from the practitioner by placing them in a system that determines what is to be done. For example, many contemporary public school teachers are disgruntled because their decisions concerning what is to be taught and how it is to be taught are being determined by pedagogical theories. Teachers are then judged not by how well they teach students or by what is learned but by how well they "teach to the task." This misuse of theory is popular with bureaucrats because it makes it possible to exert control from a central office. One reason that experienced nurses have been slow to adopt the use of nursing care plans, for example, is that it robs them of their identity by using theoretical systems to determine what they will do rather than allowing them to make decisions as competent practitioners.

Nurses and teachers are not alone in having their identity threatened by applied science. Gadamer (1981), in fact, thinks that the loss of personal identity in contemporary culture stems from our tendency to turn decision making over to specialists who make authoritative pronouncements from outside the situation. Unfortunately, contemporary nursing theory has been plagued with theories imported from outside of nursing practice. Some of the theories have been drawn from the natural sciences and others from the behavioral sciences, but whatever the source, this approach tends to separate theory from practice. Gadamer contends that "the separation of theory from practice entailed in the modern notion of the theoretical science and practical-technical application" needs to be abandoned in favor of hermeneutics which takes "the opposite path leading from practice toward making it aware of itself theoretically." (p. 131). Thus, instead of importing theories from outside in an attempt to prescribe nursing, nursing scholars, if they follow Gadamer, would engage in an interpretive articulation of the meaning of nursing as it is practiced.

The integral relationship between practice and the good in Gadamer's interpretation of practice is made evident in MacIntyre's (1984) definition of practice.

> By a "practice" I am going to mean any coherent and complex
> form of socially established cooperative human activity
> through which goods internal to that form of activity are real-
> ized in the course of trying to achieve those standards of excel-
> lence which are appropriate to, and partially definitive of, that
> form of activity, with the result that human powers to achieve
> excellence, and human conceptions of the ends and good in-
> volved, are systematically extended. (p. 187)

A practice, as MacIntyre defines it, consists primarily of whole systems of meanings and not of the particular skills involved in a practice. He contends that "bricklaying is not a practice; architecture is. Planting turnips is not a practice; farming is" (p. 187). Obviously, nursing fits within MacIntyre's definition of practice.

In contrast to those who believe that practices can be understood through theories taken from outside practice, MacIntyre (1984) contends that the goods inherent in a practice can only be understood as a part of the tradition which constitutes the practice. He rejects those who believe in outside neutral objective assessment, because he believes that excellence can only be recognized and judged by those who participate in a practice. Furthermore, any judgment concerning the worth of a practice must include its contribution both to the good of others and to the good of the practitioners themselves. Therefore, the contention that nurses should be so self-sacrificing that they neglect their own well being would, for MacIntyre, be nonsensical, because if nursing were a healthy practice, caring for others would be done in a way that fosters the well being and sense of positive identity of the nurses giving care.

According to MacIntyre, for most moderns, "the concept of a practice with goods internal to itself" has been "removed to the margins" of their lives (p. 227). Rather than placing their faith in the particular inherent goods sought through practice, they place their faith in efficient techniques and institutions. Although he recognizes that both techniques and institutions are needed to support practice, MacIntyre contends that when either becomes dominant, the good of the practice is replaced by preoccupation with correct methodology or institutional advancement as an end in itself. If nurses followed MacIntyre, they would focus on fostering the good of the patient through the practice of nursing rather than on proper methodology or institutional efficiency.

Technology is focused on efficiency. Efficiency is the "*one* value which dominates the totality of technological thought," according to Strasser (1985), because technology is "the science of the means as such" (p. 61). But "the evaluation of the efficiency of a means depends on the end which should be reached." However, "it is impossible to specify in a universally valid manner the criteria which are decisive for the evaluation of technical means" (p. 62). For example, medical science can keep a fetus alive under conditions that were formerly impossible, but it cannot judge whether a fetus with limited prospects of a normal life should be kept alive. Nor can it evaluate the often tragic consequences for the family who must care for an abnormal child with severely limited prospects for living, much less for living a meaningful life.

Benner (1984) shows how focusing on efficient knowledge derived from theoretical scientific knowledge blinds us to practical knowledge. For her, practical knowledge means "that knowledge that accrues over time" (p. 1) from actual practice. Although practical knowledge requires efficiency, efficiency in nursing practice is integrally related to the good sought in caring relationships. In Benner's descriptions of exemplars, there is no separation of ends and means. Her descriptions are devoid of a logic which says, "In order to achieve this objective, I use this means." In all of them, the technical, the personal, the relational, and the moral are integrally related to each other. These caring relationships do foster the well being of the patient but not as means to ends, as the following example indicates.

> I was taking care of a 40-year-old female who had been hospitalized for 3 months in another hospital and came to our hospital the day before to have her abdominal fistulas corrected. The night before I met her, the bag collecting her fistula drainage fell off three times and was reapplied the same way each time by her nurse due to the patient's insistence that nothing else works. Her skin was very excoriated in spots and was very tender. She was upset that nothing was working and was afraid to move because of the drainage increasing with activity. I removed the leaking bag and saw that the problem was that she had a large crease between two recessed fistulas. She was resistant to my suggestions, so I told her that she should trust me because I've had numerous similar situations

that I've had positive outcomes with. She said, "You mean you've seen a mess like this before?" This bad?," and I told her that that was our specialty here and that I was sure I could get a bag to stay on her for at least 24 hours, if not more. She said she'd love it to happen and said I could do what I wanted. She questioned all of my actions and was a bit resistant to a few suggestions and changes that I made, but I was persistent and acted very confidently about my success with such cases. I would use stomahesive paste to fill in her crevices and she'd say: "It never worked before." Then she'd say I was using too much, and I'd say that's probably why it never worked before—they never used enough. She was questioning a lot and as a result she learned a lot about the application of the appliance—specific to her. I encouraged her participation. The bag remained on for 3 days and was removed to check out the skin underneath. When we reapplied the appliance, she participated in cutting out her pattern, suctioning the drainage while we aired her skin. She actually did a lot. Her skin improved and she felt better about the situation.

I think that my confidence and insistence were the key in her acceptance of my technique. I never really doubted that I could make it work and I feel I communicated it to her and felt that giving her all of the information that I had about the procedure, step by step, that her attention was redirected positively and constructively and made her more receptive. By my taking the role of teacher she became the "student" so to speak, and that gave me the control I needed and eliminated a power struggle with her. She also became a participant in her care and had some control over her situation with her information. (pp. 130–131)

We deliberately selected this exemplar because it concerns technique and seems to employ a means-ends strategy. But notice how different it is from the means-ends strategy employed in technological interpretations of nursing. The nurse wants the patient to use her technique. But why? She has confidence that it will make the bag stay in place for an extended time as wanted by both nurse and patient. She states that her confidence led the patient to accept her technique. But can a sincere expression of confidence born of years of experience be correctly labelled as a means to an end? She also states that she gained the control she needed by assuming the role of a teacher. But can this complex intersubjective relationship between nurse and patient be adequately described as means to an end? The nurse does not teach the patient to care for herself as a means to the end of gaining control. She applies the dressing in a way that helps the patient to learn to care for her own wound. In this case, it makes no sense to talk about ends and means because the end and the means are the same—the care of the patient. In nursing, what the technological approach calls ends and means are so integrally related in actual care that they cannot be separated from each other. Significantly, this unity of ends and means is inherent in a caring practice.

THE REFORM OF NURSING PRACTICE

Reform of nursing practice might seem to be a problem for those who interpret nursing as a practice enlightened by the philosophies of practice of Gadamer and MacIntyre. Their stress on traditional practice would seem to commit nursing to maintaining the status quo. In contrast, stress on scientific technology would seem to call for rapid change in nursing because it has little or no allegiance to tradition and often regards tradition as something to be overcome. Since technology has no allegiance to tradition, it can posit any end to be sought by any means that would achieve it. Thus, it could posit ends and use means which would make nurses merely technicians who were only nominally nurses. If this occurred, how would these "nurses" be distinguished from other medical technicians. In all probability they would become general technicians who served the technical needs of physicians in giving everyday care. Thus, they would become the RCTs (registered care technicians) so much desired by the American Academy of Medicine and so much contested by the major national nursing organizations.

In contrast to a technological approach to nursing, a philosophy of practice approach would commit nurses to begin with their own practice and its inherent goods rather than with theories and models external to the practice of nursing. But this does not imply commitment to preserving the past practice intact. In fact, MacIntyre (1984) contends that a practice which is static is dead and that a live practice is a "historically extended, socially embodied argument . . . about the goods which constitute that tradition" (p. 222). This argument concerns both how the good is achieved in the practice and what the good ought to be. A live tradition does not cling to the ways of the past but instead is alive to "those future possibilities which the past has made available to the present" (p. 223). If nursing followed MacIntyre, then, it would not seek reform through importing outside procedures and methodologies, but would focus on developing and extending the goods inherent in nursing practice by recognizing and realizing the possibilities already present in its traditional practice of caring.

Rather than reforming nursing by realizing new possibilities in practice, as advocated by MacIntyre and Gadamer, technological reform regards tradition as something to be overcome with new methodologies. These new methodologies are developed by using a means-ends strategy which justifies the means used by the ends sought. Consequently, the means employed are not constrained by the discipline of the practice with its inherent good. Lack of such restraints often leads to power struggles. For example, in the struggle between the advocates of craft technology and scientific technology, the reasons given by the proponents of each position may not reflect accurately their motivations. Critical theory has made us aware that theoretical arguments often mask power struggles. For example, if nursing becomes applied theory, then theoreticians in the academy have a subtle but powerful control over nursing practice by being able to prescribe it from the academy. Nursing scholars in the academy who favor theoretical prescription of practice often interpret resistance to their prescriptions as conformity to the present power structure dominated by physicians and hospital bureaucrats. But this tendency to attack the enemy outside nursing often masks a major struggle for the control of nursing from within nursing itself. This struggle between the theoreticians in the academic world, who would prescribe nursing practice, and nursing bureaucrats, who advocate craft technology as a means of continuing bureaucratic domination, continues to this day. Interpreting nursing as the practice of caring challenges interpretations of nursing that advocate control of nursing practice either by theoretical prescription or bureaucratic mandate.

If the only alternatives for the control of nursing are believed to be theoretical prescription supported by scientific technology or bureaucratic mandate supported by craft technology, it is understandable why some nursing scholars could view an interpretation of nursing as a practice as an affirmation of the current system. For example, a critic of our recent book, when it was still in manuscript, charged us with taking a stance of appeasement and accommodation in spite of our contention that a practice is dead if it is not changing both in its understanding of the good sought and how the good is fostered. She criticized us for envisioning a form of hospital care that affirms the status quo. Her criticism entails a logic that contends that hospitals must be reformed before nursing practice can be effectively changed. In contrast, a philosophy of practice fosters change by seeking possibilities within current practice and realizing them. But who would recognize and realize these possibilities? In a philosophy of practice, scholars, rather than theoretically prescribing practice, would work with practitioners to help them recognize and realize new possibilities for excellent practice. Thus, our contention that nursing is a practice logically aligns us with Benner (1984) who believes that the reform of nursing care should be brought about by clinical nurses who give excellent innovative care to patients. In this view, authority comes from excellent practice rather than from either theoretical prescription or bureaucratic control.

In a philosophy of practice, excellent practice does not mean merely continuing current practice, however competently, but obligates practitioners to reform that practice and expand its legitimate authority whenever fostering patient well being requires it. This view of reform seems slow and tedious when compared to the prospect of rapid change by theoretical prescription from the academy or autocratic pronouncements from the managerial elite. However, most recent reforms in nursing have been achieved by changing practice from within rather than from the radical surgery prescribed by those who impatiently demand immediate change. Nurses have reformed practiced by implementing patient teaching in almost all health care settings. Nurses have taken up the slack in rural and urban health care by preparing nurse practitioners to expand nursing beyond traditional practice. Incorporating physical assessment skills by nurse practitioners made other nurses aware that they also could enhance their practice with physical assessment skills. Now these skills are practiced by many professional nurses who are not nurse practitioners. The movement to primary care also was an attempt to improve the nursing care of patients. Primary care, as originally proposed, gave a professional nurse 24-hour responsibility for a group of patients. In actual practice, however, improved care came primarily through nurses innovatively adapting the principle of primary nursing care to fit their particular situation. The above reforms are merely a few examples of how nursing practice has gradually changed by recognizing and realizing possibilities for better nursing care from within nursing practice. The effect of gradual reform on nursing practice often is overlooked by those who believe that nursing can only be reformed by theoretical prescription.

Those who favor reform by theoretical prescription also often neglect change brought about by individuals who take courageous action which, as Martin Buber (1965) puts it, ventilates the system. We encountered an excellent example of ventilating the system in a study we conducted of the experience of integration of black nurses and teachers in Virginia during the late 1960's (Scudder & Bishop, 1988). A black public health nurse requested that, rather than having her write about her experience, we grant her an extended interview. Her reason for desiring the interview was that without dialogue she was sure we would not grasp the reason for her contention that the integration of health care had not fundamentally changed her experience of being a public health nurse. She began her career long before integration was mandated by the national government. From the beginning she assumed that patients would respond to excellent nursing care. Although she was originally assigned only to black patients as her patient load, the situation in her public health assignment necessitated giving nursing care to white patients in various situations. Some white patients responded to her excellent nursing care by asking that they be assigned to her. Eventually, her nursing assignment was well integrated long before integration became mandated by law. It is hard to imagine bleaker prospects for anyone to integrate nursing practice than for a black nurse in Virginia before integration was legally mandated. And yet this nurse was able to bring integration about by giving excellent nursing care.

Some young "radical" black reformers might call this nurse an "Uncle Tom." After all, she accepted the situation as she found it and worked within it rather than attempting to reform the system. She apparently did not find it necessary to wrest her autonomy from those in control, but assumed that her deep sense of her own worth and her competence would make self-direction possible. She was able to foster local reform by ventilating the system. Those who fail to grasp this could charge her with accommodation and appeasement. However, this charge would seem strange against someone whose self-respect and competent practice established her professional autonomy in a system which denied it on the basis of race. What is remarkable about this nurse is that she extended her care into an area considered illegitimate by her society at the time, namely professional care by blacks for whites. Since then, the Civil Rights Act has made her exceptional care legitimate and expected. Of course, reforms that grant and extend legitimate authority are necessary. But expanding authority is wasted effort if that authority is not used by courageous, competent, informed and innovative nurses.

Reform is not an end in itself but should aim at freeing and encouraging excellent practitioners to improve their care of patients. Throughout this book we argue for freeing nursing practice from that type of theory that attempts to prescribe practice rather than articulate it. A theory which articulates practice enlightens practitioners so that they have the understanding necessary to adequately direct their own care of patients individually and collectively.

Innovative and collective nursing care requires that nurses free themselves from bureaucratic as well as theoretical domination. The Professional Practice Unit in the OB/GYN department at Orlando General Hospital that has developed as "an independent unit which operates all aspects, including budget, as if it were a separate hospital or private business" (*Florida Nursing News*, 1988, p. 11) offers a pertinent example of nurses freeing themselves from bureaucratic domination. The clinical nursing manager of obstetrics in that hospital reports, "Now we have autonomy. . . . We participate in decision making and there is better communication with doctors and among staff members" (p. 11). Interestingly, because of the nurses' increased self-direction, the new structure for the most part eliminated the need for the clinical nurse manager. This participant direction of nursing care logically follows from our contention that nursing is a practice and that practitioners should control nursing practice. It illustrates how nursing practice can be reformed by realizing possibilities inherent in nursing practice itself.

Again, our major contention is this: Reforms should come from realizing possibilities within the practice of nursing, rather than from restructuring nursing as a science or technology by importing theories from outside nursing practice. This does not mean, of course, that we favor rigid traditionalism. In fact, from the point of view of our philosophy of practice, a rigid traditionalism implies that practice is dead. Far from being dead, the current self-criticism in both the practice and the discipline of nursing indicates a groping and growing, live and lively practice.

THE DISTORTION OF PRACTICE THROUGH TECHNOLOGICAL REFORM

In attempting to reform nursing, nursing scholars sometimes inadvertently distort nursing practice by adopting the objective way of thinking inherent in science and applied science. Valuing the objective thought of medical science has led some nurses to lose sight of the meaning of care inherent in traditional nursing practice. Nowhere is this more evident than in the nursing diagnosis movement, whose adherents, while adopting many of the procedures and the terminology of medical science, still differentiate the movement from medical practice. By examining the treatment of hopelessness and the use of intervention language in the nursing diagnosis movement, however, we will show the effect of objective thinking on traditional values in nursing.

Most advocates of the nursing diagnosis movement believe that it will succeed in divorcing nursing from medicine because nursing diagnosis is done by nurses and is applied to nursing practice. They seem to recognize neither that the basic way of thinking in nursing diagnosis has been copied from medical science nor what effect this objective way of thinking is likely to have on nursing practice. The development of nursing diagnosis has been modeled after the International Classification of Diseases (ICD) used by physicians and health organizations all over the world. In fact, the list of nursing diagnoses which have been "approved" for use by the North American Nursing Diagnosis Association (NANDA), the official nursing diagnosis organization, has recently been revised to fit the standards and format of the ICD, and NANDA hopes to have nursing diagnoses included as part of the next revision of the ICD. Nurses who believe that nursing diagnosis will free them from medicine neglect the probable effect on nursing care of the objectifying tendencies in diagnosis.

The diagnosis of hopelessness offers a particularly revealing perspective on the effect of objectifying thought in the nursing diagnosis movement. Since hopelessness has no meaning apart from hope, it seems odd that anyone would try to treat it apart from hope. Yet, the treatment of hopelessness in one of the leading diagnostic manuals (Carpenito, 1989) is divorced from any consideration of hope. This is apparently done in order to treat hopelessness in a manner similar to the diseases diagnosed in medicine. Hopelessness, however, is not a disease or disease-like. It is, in fact, the absence of hope. Practicing nurses well know that hope is essential to patient well being and therefore fundamental in nursing care. A most frustrating experience for a nurse is caring for someone in a comatose state for whom there is no hope. Another frustration for nurses is treating patients who regard their situation as hopeless when, in fact, there is hope for a better life. Hope is so important for both nurses and patients that it has always been integral to nursing care.

How is it possible to treat hopelessness apart from hope? According to one nursing diagnosis manual, a nurse would recognize a patient who is experiencing hopelessness in the following manner. First, he or she would assess the patient to see if he or she exhibited the defining characteristics of hopelessness as given in the diagnostic manual. The nurse would recognize hopelessness by the presence of its major defining characteristics such as the expression of profound apathy, slowed responses to stimuli, passiveness, decreased verbalization, lack of ambition, and decreased problem solving (Carpenito, 1989, p. 431). Then, having determined that the patient was suffering from hopelessness, he or she would choose from a list of suggested interventions those which would "cure" hopelessness.

It is hard to imagine anyone, much less an experienced nurse, going through the above procedure to diagnose hopelessness. An experienced nurse would recognize hopelessness from vast experience of people the nurse had cared for in the past who had lost hope. The nurse would not assume, as the above description seems to, that hopelessness is a disease similar to strep throat, in that it can be objectively diagnosed in the conclusive manner that strep throat can be by using the rapid strep test. Hopelessness is not a thing but refers to the loss of hope. Since loss of hope is related to a person's outlook on life, to their situation, to their personal relationships and to many other factors, it is impossible to diagnose it as a disease-like thing, much less one thing. Hopelessness can be recognized but it cannot be objectively diagnosed.

The arid, sterile, objective description of hopelessness in the diagnostic manual is evident in the way that it deals with the time aspect of hopelessness. According to the manual, a person who is hopeless "deals with past and future, not here and now" (Carpenito, 1989, p. 432). Obviously this interpretation of hopelessness points to a tendency to live in the past or future rather than taking needed action in the present. Unfortunately, this objective way of thinking separates hopelessness from hope. Hope, after all, is primarily directed toward an anticipated future. Thus, the primary meaning of hopelessness is the inability to anticipate a desirable future. For example, a craftsman who must work with his or her body has a bleak future when a back injury has made such bodily movement impossible. His or her sense of hopelessness is fostered by memories of past satisfaction from exercising his or her talent in creating beautiful and useful cabinets. Heidegger (1962), in *Being and Time*, makes the connection between future, past, and present very clear. He interprets human being as pushing towards a projected future, drawing on a lived past, and making choices in the present that actualize future possibilities. People experience hopelessness when they can see no acceptable future possibilities. One primary meaning of illness is that one's ability to project oneself into the future in desired ways is temporarily or permanently altered. This human aspect of health care is lost when fundamental aspects of being human are objectified by treating them categorically as disease, thereby, losing the human meaning of illness. Nurses must deal with hopelessness as a response to illness or treatment, but hopelessness is not a thing to be categorized as a disease and treated by so-called interventions.

The so-called interventions in the manual (a term taken from objective scientific medicine) are not interventions at all but ways that nurses have found helpful in caring for patients who have lost hope as the following examples will indicate.

1. Listen to and treat the person as an individual.
2. Convey empathy to promote verbalization of doubt, fears, and concerns.

3. Validate and reflect impressions with the person.
4. Encourage family to express their love and need for the person.

(Carpenito, 1989, pp. 439–440)

These suggestions should be useful in helping patients recover hope, but does it make sense to refer to them as interventions? Intervention means to intervene in something. According to Edmund Pellegrino (1985), interventions in medical care concern "the natural history of the disease" (p. 12). Therefore, intervention suggests an activity such as terminating an infection with a shot of penicillin. Imagine terminating hopelessness with a shot of hope!

The inadequacy of treating hopelessness as a thing to be diagnosed and treated by intervention can be shown by interpreting the following example of a patient experiencing hopelessness as a result of being confined to a nursing home.

> *Well, here's* another *day . . . I'll swear, how slowly they pass . . . and you wonder why I can't be cheerful about things. . . . I'm trying, I really am tryin', but I'm not gettin' anywhere . . . When he [her pulmonary specialist] told me that there wasn't any possible chance for me to get out and have another apartment on my own . . . and . . . that I'd always have to live in a place like this . . . that . . . that did somethin' to me . . . I really couldn't shake it. . . . I know I'm gloomy and sad, an' all that. You'll just have to bear with me. . . . I may get used to it, an' I may not . . . 'ts a bad deal. . . . (Zaner, 1988, p. 268)*

Obviously, those who were caring for the above patient had conveyed to her that she should respond to her situation by being happy and content. Why should she be unhappy and discontent? After all, she only faces the actuality of living the rest of her life in a place and situation she finds intolerable. If her nurses are to help her find possibilities and hence hope, they must do so by helping her discover and realize the possibilities within her actual situation of being ill in the nursing home.

Her hopelessness is not merely the consequence of her illness, however, but also results from the kind of nursing care she is receiving, as she makes evident.

*I know . . . [clears throat] . . . I know that no matter . . .
how long my sentence is . . . it's gonna be spent in a nursing
home, alone. . . . Can't think of a worse way to spend it
th' . . . than in a nursing home. Which is just like bein' in
jail, really. You have no rights; you're just a number. A baby.
An' all the bodies are old and worn out, an' yours is no
different than anybody else's. . . . An' I found that it's not
any advantage at all . . . to have your . . . brains left, because, when you question things, they think you're trying to tell
them how to run their business. . . . It's better not to question, it's better just t' go 'n accept their discipline like a child
would.* (Zaner, 1988, p. 268)

Obviously, one reason she feels hopeless is that her self-direction has
been taken from her. Facing the remainder of her life in a nursing
home away from her family is depressing enough without having to
deny that she's "got brains." Obviously, the first step in restoring hope
to this patient would be to allow her to use her "brains" in assuming
the maximum possible self-direction. This would help restore hope to
her because of the kind of person she is. Being made dependent is
abhorrent to this patient. She is a very self-directing person who finds
losing self-care to be a prison sentence. How strange it would be to call
allowing this person to direct her own life as much as possible an
intervention. In her case, the intervention would be in the nursing care
she is receiving. Nurses who use contemporary objectifying language
often call all that they do to and for patients interventions. Such
objective language as intervention obscures the human meaning of
illness. Obviously, it is illness that has intervened in this person's life as
she has been accustomed to live it and wants to live it, namely, inde-
pendently. Furthermore, her nurses are intervening in her life by not
allowing her to use her brains. Does she need an intervention to
remove that intervention? Such confusion in language as the foregoing
results from using objective language inappropriately. Intervention in
medical language is used appropriately when it means that some medical procedure has intervened in the natural course of a disease; for
example, penicillin intervening in the course of a disease called strep
throat. But hopelessness is not a disease and thus cannot be objectively
defined and eliminated with intervention. Hopelessness has no meaning apart from hope; it is the absence of hope. Hope has to do with

anticipated future. Illness and debilitation threaten a person's anticipated future, thus fostering hopelessness. Recovering hope has to do
with discovering possibilities of a satisfactory life for particular persons
in certain circumstances. Does it make any sense to designate as an
intervention the activity of helping someone find possibilities for a
good life?

Our purpose in raising this issue is not to foster semantic purity.
Instead, we are concerned with the possible consequences of injecting
scientific objective terminology and thought into the practice of caring.
Nurses who have engaged in the practice of caring over the years were
well aware of the detrimental effects of hopelessness and of the positive
effects of hope on patient well being long before Norman Cousins
(1989) cited the scientific evidence for it. In fact, many nurses believe
that they are much more aware of these aspects of health care than most
physicians, because they see them at work in the day-to-day care they
give to patients. How strange that nurses should turn to the objectifying
procedures of diagnosis used by physicians in order to recognize such
fundamental human experiences as hopelessness. An artificially con-
cocted objective system of diagnosis, however necessary to receive third
party payment, seems strangely out of place in a practice created over
many years by caring for patients who, as a consequence of illness, have
lost the hope that formerly had empowered their lives.

Some advocates of the nursing diagnosis movement might say that
we have treated the movement unfairly by focusing on that aspect of
nursing diagnosis most suited to our purposes. They would be right, of
course, if our purpose had been to appraise the nursing diagnosis
movement, which we have neither the preparation nor inclination to
do. Our purpose has been to show what happens when objective ways
of thinking are inappropriately imported into nursing care. We chose
to examine hopelessness not because it is the most typical example of
nursing diagnosis but because it showed how importing the objectifying procedures of medical science into a caring practice reduces a
fundamental aspect of human being into a thing-like disease. In so
doing, it needlessly complicates and distorts the nursing care of those
who have lost hope as a consequence of illness.

It is regretable that traditional nursing practice, which has been so
amenable to incorporating such human values as hope into its care,
should de-emphasize these values by restructuring itself with objective
thought. This is especially unfortunate at a time when even medicine is

becoming more aware of the contribution of human values and aspirations to healing and recovery. An outstanding group of medical researchers at UCLA are reversing the negative meaning of the psychosomatic in medicine ("it's all in your head") by experimentally proving that faith, love, and hope actually enhance the immune system (Cousins, 1989). At a time when the human meaning of healing and wellness is coming to the fore, nursing, given its caring tradition, should seek to realize the possibilities inherent in nursing practice for further developing those human meanings essential to good health.

APPROPRIATE MEDICAL SCIENCE
IN NURSING CARE

Our opposition to restructuring nursing from a caring practice to a technology should not be construed as opposition to the use of medical science and technology in nursing practice. There is a great difference between a caring practice that uses technology and a caring practice that is structured as a technology. (In fact, one could question the appropriateness of calling an activity structured as a technology a caring practice.) Much of the improvement in health care since World War II has come from advances in medical science and technology. These improvements have been mixed blessings, however, as nurses well know who wrestle with the problem of caring for irreversibly comatose patients or for premature babies kept alive only to suffer and cause suffering for their parents until their death. Despite the many difficulties that medical science and technology have created, however, their overall contribution to health care seems unquestionable. In fact, much of the recent development in the caring tradition that is nursing has involved incorporating medical science and technology into nursing practice. Gadow (1985) well recognizes this problem in her contention that contemporary nurses must be able to treat the body object without objectifying the person. Although she believes the use of modern technology often fosters objectification of the patient, she contends that the primary source of objectifying patients is interpreting nursing as a technology.

The primary threat to nursing practice is not the use of science and technology but interpreting nursing as an applied science. Viewing nursing as a caring practice with an inherent moral aim does not necessarily favor one particular style of nursing over another. Modern high-tech intensive care nurses are no less engaged in a caring practice than older style nurses who gave direct care. Nurses who work in critical care units and like the challenge of working in high-tech areas are viewed by some nurses as having abandoned the traditional practice of caring. But those who make such charges regard an older style of nursing care as nursing itself, neglecting the fact that nursing practice is a developing tradition that changes in order to better foster patient well being. One cutting edge of that tradition involves using medical science and technology to foster patient well being while maintaining a personal caring relationship between nurse and patient. How the meaning of this development can be misunderstood is indicated by the response of participants in a nursing conference to the results of an interest inventory given to intensive care nurses. Since nurses in intensive care units need to like and be proficient in medical technology, it did not surprise attending nurses that intensive care nurses scored high on the mechanical and scientific areas of an interest inventory. Their low scores on the nurturing/altruism items, however, caused considerable concern to the nurses attending the conference. They perceived these results as a threat to the future of nursing, since they believed that nursing would make increasingly greater use of technology. But their apprehension may well have been, in part, unwarranted. Nursing style is often confused with the meaning and purpose of nursing. Nurses can care for the well being of patients with a highly technological style as well as a very personal and direct style. For example, an intensive care nurse described her patient who had undergone an aneurysm clipping as "a GCS5T, E4 M1, VT [who] opened his eyes but [had] no movement and was trached." It is obvious from this description that this nurse worked in a highly technical situation. She abandoned her technological language when she expressed her feelings concerning the outcome of her nursing care. "I can't describe the sensation I felt; but to see him follow a command for the first time— moving his thumb made me feel wonderful inside. All our diligent nursing care, positioning, ROM, stimulation, etc. was working and it felt good" (Bishop & Scudder, 1990, pp. 99–100). The elation that came from seeing a thumb move involved understanding a whole complex system of nursing care. But when the nurse expressed her delight at the outcome of this complex care, it was given as an expression of personal feeling. Significantly, this nurse said that although she liked working with complex technology, she would not continue in nursing if it were not for the fulfillment which came from the moral and personal sense of nursing. Obviously, she had incorporated high technology into traditional nursing practice by caring for her patient, both in the sense of caring for his well being and in giving him excellent care.

The nurse in the foregoing example was fulfilling her moral responsibility as a nurse. The first and foremost moral responsibility of a nurse is excellent practice. Often the moral significance of excellent practice is missed by those who believe that good moral action is recognized only by its conformity to the traditional way in which philosophers have made moral judgements. Following this procedure, a nurse when confronted by some moral problem would decide what to do by following the dictates of a moral norm, such as utilitarianism or autonomy. But in the above case, the nurse was not confronted with a moral problem. Instead, she was concerned about the well being of the patient, used sound nursing practice to foster his well being, and determined by the movement of his thumb that his well being was being fostered. Sound nursing practice has an integral moral sense that fosters the good of the patient by excellent nursing care. Consequently, the first moral responsibility of the nurse is excellent care.

The profession of nursing is committed to giving excellent care; the above case being an exemplar of such care. However, the meaning of care exemplified in this case is very different from the meaning given to professional care by the advocates of scientific technological nursing. According to the scientific-technological interpretation, a person becomes a professional by possessing the special knowledge and skill which sets him or her apart from those not in the profession. Then commitment to use this knowledge and skill for the benefit of others is added on to the scientific-technical meaning of profession. In contrast to this add-on interpretation of profession, Pellegrino (1985) contends that the primary meaning of profession is moral in that it comes from professing to do good for the patient. But meeting the moral demands of such a profession does require the knowledge and skill necessary to fulfill what is professed. The nursing excellences discussed by Benner (1984) are descriptions of how the moral profession of nurses is fulfilled through nursing knowledge and skill. The moral profession of nursing also is fulfilled by the in-between stance that makes possible the daily care that fosters the well being of patients. In both cases, the knowledge and skill used are integrally related to patient well being. This implies that the moral sense of nursing care is not an add-on to nursing knowledge and skill. Instead, care names the way of fostering the good of a patient through a nurse–patient relationship empowered by concern for the well being of the patient and by knowledge and skill. Care names the inherent good of nursing practice integrally related to the way in which it is sought and the relationship through which it is given.

4

Nursing as Caring

In contrast to the integral relationship of care as the good fostered and care as the way in which it is fostered, care is often interpreted as an inner feeling of beneficence detached from concrete taking care of others. Disclaiming that this inner meaning of care was the primary meaning of nursing obviously was the target of the following television advertisement: "If you have the smarts and the guts to study biology, chemistry, anatomy and psychology . . . call 1-800-962-NURSE. If caring were enough, anyone could be a nurse." These words were accompanied by visuals that showed nurses intensely engaged in caring for patients in an obvious emergency situation. Doubtless, those who sponsored the above advertisement wanted to recruit new nurses by making the claim that being a nurse involves more than being a well-meaning person who is concerned for the ill and debilitated. Unfortunately in achieving this commendable goal, caring is treated as an inner feeling divorced from the concrete giving of care. Thus this advertisement depreciates the practice of nursing and conveys an inaccurate conception of what constitutes both nursing and caring.

The inadequate grasp of the meaning of caring implied in the television advertisement is understandable, given a culture like ours that still suffers the Cartesian dualism between mind and body. Those who work from this philosophical assumption regard caring as an inner "subjective" feeling—if caring were enough, anyone could be a nurse. The advertisement also implies that what sets nurses apart from mere caring persons is not that they have mastered the practice of nursing care but that they have studied biology, chemistry, anatomy, and psychology. In other words, nursing is significant because nurses apply science and not merely because they care. After all, anyone can care.

Obviously, some nurses do not believe it is as easy to care for others as the advertisement implies. If it were, it is difficult to explain why some thoughtful nurses attending an ethics conference asked us, "Is it not possible to give good nursing care without caring personally for each patient?" What raised this question was our attempt to interpret nursing ethics in light of various philosophies of caring. We responded to their question by pointing out that nurses need not have a warm, inner, beneficent feeling toward each patient in order to give adequate nursing care. However, it is difficult to imagine anyone giving good nursing care if he or she were not concerned about the patient's well being. Caring is a relational term that has two meanings: concern for others and taking care of others. In nursing, care signifies both concern for the well being of others and taking care of them. It would make no sense for a nurse to say, "I am concerned for the well being of my patients, but I am not taking care of them." A nurse expresses his or her concern for the ill by giving excellent nursing care regardless of whether or not he or she likes the patient as a person. When it is put this way, the worth of nursing comes neither from having inner beneficent feelings toward the ill nor from applying such sciences as anatomy, psychology, chemistry, and biology to nursing practice. Nursing is a significant enterprise because it is a practice through which human concern for the well being of ill and debilitated persons is concretely expressed through expert nursing care.

The television advertisement not only distorts caring by making it an inner feeling divorced from concrete care, but it distorts nursing practice itself. Active concrete caring for ill persons requires a way of caring. The way of caring of a nurse is not the same as anyone who cares for the ill, except for a few mundane activities. What makes the nurse's way of caring different from anyone else's is not that nurses have taken a few science courses. (Scudder, in the course of becoming a philosopher, has taken more than a smattering of science courses, but it is hard to imagine him giving professional nursing care). Nurses are different from amateurs caring for the ill in that they have appropriated and mastered the caring practice of nursing.

Persons outside of nursing who have some knowledge of nursing practice might find it difficult to understand why nurses value their practice so little that they would seek to establish its importance by attaching it to taking science courses in college. This lack of appreciation for practice is evident in the claim that nurses show their "guts" by taking elementary courses in science. Scudder, for example, seriously questioned whether or not he has "the guts" to care for patients in the way actually shown in the television advertisement which makes the odd claim that it takes guts to take science courses. In contrast to the guts required to take introductory science courses, compare Sallie Tisdale's (1986) vivid description of the tenuous balance required in nursing practice.

> *Somewhere in this trial is a middle way, a balance of pain and compassion. Burn nurses find it or quit. It is a narrow trail flanked by extremity. One side, the side of empathy, is filled with wrenching sorrow, anger, and despair. It is where another person's pain becomes so visible, so inarguably present, that we attempt to take it on as we might carry a burden. . . .*
>
> *On the other side is a kind of total severance from the person in pain. This is more than detachment—it is actually a fissure within the person not in pain from his or her own memory and experience. (p. 129)*

Nurses need "guts", then, not in order to take elementary science courses but to give nursing care.

Not only is it difficult for a non-nurse like Scudder to understand why nurses would make the claim that they show their "guts" by taking introductory science courses, it is equally difficult for him to understand why taking these courses demonstrates their "smarts." Of course, one has to be moderately intelligent to pass a science course. But much more intelligence is required to appropriate a complex practice like nursing in a way that expresses the nurse's personal way of being in giving care that is appropriate to a particular patient in a given situation.

We have criticized the advertisement concerning nursing not because it is a serious treatment of nursing but in order, through contrast, to make the point that nursing is a caring practice which has its own worth. It need not borrow its significance from the natural sciences. True, nurses need to know some science in order to practice, but they show their "smarts" and "guts" in the exercise of their caring practice.

CARING AS A WAY OF BEING: HEIDEGGER

Heidegger's (1962) ontological interpretation of caring as a fundamental human way of being-in-the-world stands in sharp contrast to those, like the authors of the television advertisement, who regard caring as some inner beneficent feeling separated from the world. In his famous work, *Being and Time*, Heidegger persuasively shows that caring is a fundamental, if not *the* fundamental, way of being for humans. A human being is that being who must care for self and for others. The implications of Heidegger's interpretation of care for nursing can be made evident by considering the essential meaning of becoming mature. A mature person is one who can care for self and others in a given cultural context. This accomplishment in primitive societies takes 12 to 14 years but in complex, developed societies 20 years or more. A great deal of parenting and schooling is aimed precisely at preparing persons to care for themselves and others. It is necessary to care for the young because they cannot adequately care for themselves. Care also becomes necessary for the old and the ill and debilitated when they cannot care for themselves without the help of others.

AUTHENTIC CARING

Caring for others is necessary when they are unable to care for themselves. The necessity for such care gives the caregiver much power over the person receiving care. Care can be given in ways that take self-direction from the one being cared for. Heidegger (1962) makes this evident by contrasting two ways of caring for others. In the first way, a person will "*leap in*" for another and "take over for the other." This form of care can readily foster domination and dependency when the caregiver "leaps in and takes away 'care'." We will call this dependent care because it fosters dependency on others. In contrast to dependent care, authentic care (so named by Heidegger) occurs when the care giver will "*leap ahead*" [ihm vorausspringt] in his existentiell (sic) potentiality-for-Being, not in order to take away his 'care' but rather to give it back to him authentically" (pp. 159–160). Thus, in authentic care the other is helped to care for his or her own being.

Heidegger (1962) helps us to understand that these two forms of caring for others have important implications for human being and becoming. Dependent care makes the individual's being and becoming dependent on others, thus threatening to take self-care from the one cared for. In contrast, authentic care attempts to restore self-care to those who have lost it due to illness or debilitation.

Authentic care also is threatened by technological thought which treats human beings as objects and prescribes their way of being. Objective categories, which are more appropriate for thinking about things rather than human beings, are used in Western language, according to Heidegger (1962), to designate human beings as static entities. Objective language places humans in categories that define them as having fixed natures. For this reason, objective language encourages static dependent care rather than that self-care which fosters human becoming through the realization of possibilities in the world.

For Heidegger, care is that which unifies actuality and possibility (Gelven, 1970, p. 74). All things exist at the level of actuality in that their being is determined by other forces. Human beings are those beings who can care for their own being because they can recognize and fulfill possibilities in their actual situation. For Heidegger, freedom means to act to fulfill possibilities that are present in actual situations. Since humans are capable of recognizing possibilities in their actual situation and have the ability, within limits, to realize them, they are beings who choose their own being by caring for their own being and the being of others.

Obviously for Heidegger (1962), authentic care is focused on future possibility and on freedom. When most Westerners think of care, they usually think of actuality rather than possibility and of beneficent control rather than freedom. It is easy to see why care is thought of as actuality and control when examining health care. After all, those who must seek help from medical and nursing experts are dependent on them for their well being. All nurses have given extreme forms of dependent care, when patients were completely unable to care for themselves. They have seen the gratitude in patient's eyes for care given. Nurses also have seen the frustration, the despair, and even hatred in the eyes of very self-directed persons who have to be waited on hand and foot as a result of serious illness. Such persons resent losing self-care even when it is necessary. Nurses know both of the necessity for dependent care and of the desire for self-care.

Nurses also know that nursing care, itself, presupposes possibility. Nursing care is given in the hope of fostering future possible well being. Having to care for someone when there is absolutely no hope makes health care seem futile. This is why caring for patients like Karen Ann Quinlan and Nancy Cruzan for whom there is no hope of recovery of human consciousness so troubles our conscience. When actuality rules out possibility, care loses much of its primary meaning.

For Heidegger (1962), the relationship of actuality and possibility is one of time. He develops this analysis of care by arguing that the primary essence of man is being in time. His interpretation of time, called "lived time," involves pushing towards a projected future while drawing on the past and making choices in the present that actualize future possibilities. Put differently, being in time involves being directed toward possibilities that grow out of actuality, the fulfillment of which requires drawing on an actual past so as to bring about present action that attempts to fulfill projected future possibilities of being. For example, some patients will choose therapy which involves enduring greater pain if this means they will recover more rapidly and will be able to leave the hospital sooner and resume their normal life. The hope of resuming their normal life calls forth the resources necessary to endure the short-term pain required for therapeutic treatment that enhances the possibility of resuming a normal life. In contrast, several nurses in the study that we (Bishop & Scudder, 1990) conducted on fulfillment in nursing in a tertiary medical center, reported to us that they felt most unfulfilled when they cared for patients who had literally no hope for improvement but were subjected to countless interventions which kept them biologically alive at the cost of "living" in pain and misery. These nurses often implied that the use of such medical interventions was dictated by the professional needs of physicians rather than the desire to help patients live as well as possible for the remainder of their lives. Also, in these cases, what the patient desired often was not considered unless one regards signing a consent form as adequate consideration of how one wants to live the remainder of his life. Fostering the well being of the patient requires bringing together in coherent action the knowledge of the actual condition of the patient, the abilities and resources of health care workers, the formulation and execution of a plan of action, and the patient's understanding of and desire for a good life in the future. When these actualities and possibilities make sense as a whole, then coherence in time is achieved, which, if we follow Heidegger, actually means that good health *care* is being given.

All patient care is founded on seeing possibilities for fostering patient well being. These possibilities can range from full recovery to limiting pain in the face of certain and painful death. In any case, the nurse's actual care of the patient grows out of the possibility the nurse sees for better patient well being. In authentic care, the nurse focuses his or her care on the possibilities for increasing the patient's self-care. Obviously, there are situations in which patients cannot take care of themselves. For example, patients immediately after major surgery cannot climb out of bed and go to the toilet. In such cases the nurse literally takes care of the patient, but this should be done only when the patients are unable to take care of themselves. However, nurses sometimes care for their patients out of their own need to care. Unfortunately, this laudable need to care for others hides a real danger. It is easy for the *need* to care to blind nurses to the possibilities for self-care. When this occurs, the nurse rather than taking care *of* the patient is actually taking care *from* the patient. When nurses take care *from* the patient, they deny the patient the possibility of the self-care that is essential to being fully human.

When nurses take care *of* patients rather than taking care *from* patients, they fulfill the moral sense of nursing by fostering the full well being of patients. The moral sense of nursing asserts the priority of possibility over actuality which, for Heidegger (1962), leads to being authentic. Inauthentic human beings give priority to actuality over possibility in that they let their past self or others dictate their actions and therefore their way of being in the world. In contrast, an authentic person chooses his or her own life from the possibilities present in his or her world.

Encouraging patients to live authentically fosters recovery and wellness. Norman Cousins (1989) has shown that a hopeful defiant spirit can overcome even biological actualities. He not only provides numerous examples of such cases but also cites scientific studies that empirically demonstrate that hope, love, and will to live actually enhance the immune system's ability to fight disease (pp. 85–87). This is the reason he subtitles his recent book, *The Biology of Hope*. He supports his thesis with many examples of how despair impairs the effectiveness of the immune system. In some cases, this impairment is fostered by the tone of finality conveyed when physicians communicate the imminence of death. Cousins, however, also provides examples of how defiant spirit can overcome such a prognosis. "'I looked him straight in the eye,' she said, 'and told him to go straight to hell. God could give me four months to live but not another human being. That was six years ago'" (p. 83).

Cousins (1989) shows how good counsel and love can foster authentic living to the end of life. A judge who "had been known for courage, determination, and a positive outlook of life" gave up fighting and withdrew into himself on being told that he would soon die of cancer. Cousins, who had been asked by the judge's physician to talk with him, gives the following account of his counsel.

> I said that Dr. Bluming had given me a briefing on his condition and that I was also concerned about his wife and sons and, in fact, about all the people who loved him.
>
> His eyes narrowed in a way that indicated he wanted me to explain myself. I said I understood that all his life he had been a fighter for things he considered just and right.
>
> He nodded and again he narrowed his eyes as though to find out what I was getting at.
>
> I said that one of the things I had learned at the medical school was that the attitude of the patient had a profound effect on members of the family. Their health could be jeopardized by negative attitudes of the patient. I said I hoped he would forgive me if I said that his family was anguished by the judge's apparent defeatism. Such defeatism might seem natural in anyone else, but in the judge . . .
>
> The judge closed his eyes momentarily. Then he looked at me and uttered just two words:
>
> "I gotcha." (pp. 23–24)

Soon after the talk, the judge began to eat, play bridge, communicate with his family and even defied the nurse's insistence that he use the bedpan. His wife vividly described the change in him.

> "The judge's spirits have been wonderful," she said. "He has had good talks with our sons. He follows the newspapers and makes his usual witty comments. He now takes walks in the hospital corridors and chats with other patients. The ultimate

outlook hasn't changed, but the general atmosphere has. We are . . . well, a lot less despondent than we were." (pp. 24–25)

Although the judge only survived several weeks, Cousins well sums up the meaning of those weeks.

> It was a magnificent example of how the human spirit could make a difference—not just in prolonging one's life but in bolstering the lives of others. The judge's deep sense of purpose didn't reverse the disease—the cancer had spread so widely to his vital organs that it was only a question of time before it would claim his life. But he was also able to govern the circumstances of his passing in a way that provided spiritual nourishment to the people who loved him. He died in character. This was his gift to everyone who knew him.
>
> Hope, faith, love, and a strong will to live offer no promise of immortality, only proof of our uniqueness as human beings and the opportunity to experience full growth even under the grimmest circumstances. (p. 25)

Nurses, because they are close to dying patients in the grimmest of circumstances and relate to patients out of a caring tradition, are uniquely suited for fostering authentic living to the end and sometimes even beyond the end predicted by medical prognosis through the biology of hope.

Authentic care not only means that nursing care should foster authentic living for patients, but it also means that nurses should care authentically. Authentic nurses choose their own way of caring for each particular patient. In contrast, inauthentic nurses let others take their care giving *from* them by letting decisions concerning that care be determined by theories, past teachers of nursing, supervisors, procedure manuals, peer pressure or even their own past selves. However, authentic nursing does not imply inventing nursing practice anew with each patient. Instead, it requires appropriating sound nursing practice into each nurse's particular way of being with particular patients.

The contention that nurses ought to give authentic care obviously states a moral imperative, even though Heidegger (1962) himself did not interpret authenticity and inauthenticity as moral issues. Indeed, the possibility of developing a Heideggerian ethic is a major problem for interpreters of Heidegger. Heidegger does, however, point ethics in the right direction by asserting the priority of possibility over actuality. After all, morality deals with what ought to be. What ought to be is what is actually not now but could be and should be. The practice of nursing itself is founded on the moral imperative that people ought to be well. Nursing practice consists of ways of fostering the physical and psychological well being of persons by caring for them when illness or debilitation make them incapable of caring for their own well being. Nursing care becomes authentic care when nurses give responding and responsible care which enhances, restores, or increases self-care to the degree possible. By so doing, patients are not merely helped to cope with illness and debilitation but are encouraged and empowered to continue their quest for full humanity.

Authentic care does not imply a self-autonomy that isolates self from others and world. Caring for self and others is always done in the world. Thus, care for persons cannot be divorced from care for the world. The phrase much used by Heidegger, *being-in-the-world*, signifies that being and world are integrally related. In contrast to Heidegger (1962), however, Westerners have traditionally separated the so-called inner subjective from the so-called outer objective world. In this artificial dichotomy, care has been placed on the intersubjective and value side and science on the objective and knowledge side. Following this dichotomy, caring has become an inner feeling which could be treated as if it were divorced from the world in which care is given. Furthermore, since objective knowledge has been valued more than subjective feeling, care has been devalued. (After all, anyone can care.) Care also has been denigrated because science and objective knowledge have tended to be regarded as masculine enterprises, whereas valuing and intersubjective knowledge have been regarded as feminine concerns. The traditional views, that knowledge and value are separate and that objective knowledge is superior to intersubjective knowledge and value, have been effectively challenged by the feminist theories of caring of Carol Gilligan (1980) and Nell Noddings (1984).

THE WEB OF CONNECTION: GILLIGAN

Gilligan (1980) contends that women reach moral maturity when they give authentic care to self and others in a web of connection. She bases her contention on psychological studies of how women actually make moral decisions in contrast to men. As Gilligan makes evident, the development of moral decision making by men had been unwittingly done by the Psychologist, Lawrence Kohlberg, (1958, 1981). Kohlberg claimed to have discovered the way in which morality develops in all human beings on the basis of examples taken only from men. Gilligan, by studying the ways in which women make moral decisions, was able to show that women generally make moral decisions differently from men.

We will treat only that part of Gilligan's (1980) interpretation that is needed to show how her theory can help us better appreciate the significance of the in-between in nursing practice. Gilligan offers a helpful distinction between the masculine and feminine in her treatment of how men and women break out of what Kohlberg (1981) designates as the conventional stage of development. According to Kohlberg, a man breaks out of the conventional stage by becoming autonomous and reflective, eventually establishing thereby abstract and universal moral principles. In contrast, according to Gilligan, a woman breaks out of the conventional stage by discovering herself and seeing the interconnection between herself and others. In this final ethical stage, a woman discovers her worth and responds by caring for self and others. This discovery of self-worth and response by caring results in a caring ethic that stresses responsible relationships. The woman's ethic of caring relationships contrasts markedly with the man's ethic which stresses formal logic, rights, and justice.

In a culture which overvalues so-called masculine virtues and devalues so-called feminine virtues, it is understandable why leaders in professions consisting primarily of women, such as nursing, would initially assert "masculine" virtues in attempting to free their professions from parameters set by men. For example, some scholars who stress the need for autonomy in nursing (Yarling & McElmurry, 1986; Foulk and Keffer, 1991) were critical of our contention that one essential way of being in nursing practice was the in-between stance of the nurse (Bishop & Scudder, 1987).

Gilligan's (1980) interpretation of caring lends support to our contention that the nurses' in-between stance is a necessary and positive stance which nurses should prize. Furthermore, she makes evident the inadequacy of over-stressing autonomy in health care. She defines caring as "an activity of relationship, of seeing and responding to need, taking care of the world by sustaining the web of connection so that no one is left alone" (p. 62). This feminine image of relationships as a web contrasts sharply with the masculine image of relationships, the hierarchical pyramid. Viewed from the image of hierarchy, the person on top is autonomous, because he or she is in control and truly self-directing. Viewed from the image of the web, however, the top of the hierarchy is peripheral and the center is focal. Those who follow the image of the hierarchy desire to be "alone at the top" where authoritative and often authoritarian decisions are made, whereas those who follow the image of the web "wish to be at the center of the connection" (p. 62) where relationships are more interconnected. When relationships are "cast in the image of hierarchy," they "appear inherently unstable and morally problematic," but when transposed into an image of web, relationships can change from "an order of inequality into a structure of interconnection" (p. 62). Maintaining this interconnection in health care has fallen almost entirely on nurses. The traditional in-between stance of the nurse is rooted in the web of connectedness. Traditionally, nurses have been called on to maintain the connection between patient, family, hospital, and physician. Such connection is not only feminine, but it is required for daily care. A nurse is not in-between by some accident of tradition but in order to *give* daily care. To do this, the nurse must be able to work with the physician, patient, family, and the hospital bureaucrat, bringing them together so as to foster good health. In our previous example of the in-between, the nurse who helped the dying patient celebrate Christmas as he desired was able to do so because she worked from the center of the web of relationships.

Gilligan (1980) helps us to see the importance of fostering the web of connectedness. Interestingly, the web of connectedness also is regarded as necessary for physicians by those interpreters of medicine who regard medicine as a caring practice, such as Pellegrino (1985), Richard Zaner (1985, 1988), and Engelhardt (1985). Although most nurses will welcome this new direction in medicine, fostering interconnectedness in health care undoubtedly will remain a primary stance of nursing, not because most nurses are women, but because the practice of giving daily care places nurses uniquely in an in-between position.

THE PATIENT IN THE WEB OF CONNECTION

Like nurses, patients also are bound together in a web of connection. For example, a nurse learned to live in a web of connection that extended far beyond hospital relationships when she had to learn to live with continuing bodily deterioration due to acute myelomonocytic leukemia. This nurse-patient organized and directed her own care in order to live as much of her remaining life as possible in normal situations outside of the hospital. She was able to do this because her understanding of health care extended far beyond hospital and nursing care to that vast network of ordinary care that often goes unnoticed. Her care also makes evident the kinds of care required when the ill are cared for at home. People seriously ill in their home require the three kinds of care evident in the following example of the above nurse's care: care given by health care professionals, care related to the world outside the home, and care in the form of interpersonal support.

When M. returned home following hospitalization, she continued to require support and monitoring of her condition. A local home health agency provided skilled personnel for drawing of necessary blood samples, changing Hickman catheter dressings, and administering intravenous medications. The questions remained, however, of who would supply emotional support and contact with the outside world? . . . .

For M., help from her comfort caregivers came in many forms. Often it was a ride to the doctor's office or the hospital for blood or platelets. On good days it was a steady arm to walk beside her as she worked to strengthen her atrophied muscles or a chance to see the new baby in the neighborhood or have lunch with tennis friends. . . . Many times the comfort came as peaceful rest periods or opportunities to cry and express feelings about life and death. . . . The greatest compliment for M. seemed to be for one of her friends to share some recent difficulty in her own life. M. offered words of comfort from her own life experiences which reassured the caregiver. The therapeutic effect on M. was a sense of being

well enough to confront with others their troubles. The loss that
M. suffered by her early retirement from a profession that was
so energizing to her was somehow lessened when she was able
to care for and comfort others. . . . (Arrington & Walborn,
1989, pp. 25–26)

The above case shows how care giving and receiving are mutual. M. received much care from friends and colleagues, but she also responded by caring for them. Although the most obvious form of her care was in the counsel she gave to friends, she also cared for them by the gracious way she received care and by being herself in the face of the pain, debilitation, and grim prospects of terminal illness. Nurses, in giving care to such persons, need to help them become aware of how much they can give to others by living authentically in the face of impending death. One nursing student expressed this well in commenting on the contribution made to her by a dying patient's way of being. "In the midst of her pain and suffering, she constantly praised everything I did for her. Just to experience the presence of a person so at peace with herself was a terrific highlight in my life" (Bishop & Scudder, 1990, p. 98).

The case of M. not only shows the importance of being (who we are) to a people who overvalue having and doing, it also shows how we are dependent on care given by others, of which we ordinarily are not aware. M.'s illness made it necessary to marshal the care that we normally take for granted in our daily living. M.'s being a nurse highlights the fact that nursing care is an important and specialized form of care. However, it is only one form of caring in that vast web of connection required for human well being.

M.'s example also shows how dependent care, when it is given in a web of connection, can become authentic care. M. had to depend on others to live as well as she did. Their care, however, rather than taking care from her, made it possible for her to care for herself as much as possible. Authentic care does not require that the patient not depend on others. Ill persons such as M. must depend on the care of others in order to care for themselves. M. learned to depend on others in a web of connection that made it possible for her to care for herself as much as she could.

NATURAL AND ETHICAL CARING: NODDINGS

Noddings (1984) develops a caring ethic in which intersubjective care fosters self-care. Her caring ethic stresses both mutuality and recognizing and fostering self-direction by the one cared for. Her caring ethic begins with natural caring which she defines as "that relationship in which we respond as one caring out of love or natural inclination" (p. 5). We will focus on how natural caring appears, thereby following accepted phenomenological methodology. By doing so, it is possible to define natural caring merely as caring which is natural to the one giving care without attributing it to organic causes. When natural caring is defined in this way, it makes sense to say that most nurses, like most parents, naturally care for those entrusted to their care.

Caring first appears, according to Noddings (1984), when "we accept the natural impulse to act on behalf of the present other" (p. 83). Beginning with the natural inclination to care, Noddings develops an ethic of caring that assumes intersubjective "relation as ontologically basic and the caring relation as ethically basic" (p. 150). Essential elements in the caring relationship include "*engrossment* and *motivational displacement* on the part of the one-caring and a form of *responsiveness* or *reciprocity* on the part of the cared-for" (p. 150).

Noddings (1984) articulates one-caring first as engrossment with another and then as motivational shift toward the other. When I am engrossed, "I receive the other into myself, and I see and feel with the other" (p. 30). I receive what the other shares without evaluation or assessment. When I care for others, my caring includes their experience of the world. How we care grows out of the "constellation of conditions that is viewed through both the eyes of the one-caring and the eyes of the cared-for" (p. 13).

An excellent example of the engrossment is given by Claire Hastings in her description of her relationship with one of her patients.

I had a powerful clinical experience when I was working in the Rheumatology Screening Clinic. . . . An older woman in a wheelchair came with her daughter. I remember that she had terrible rheumatoid arthritis. When we say "terrible

rheumatoid arthritis," we mean someone who might be presented in a textbook —one with a lot of deformities, who can't
walk and is all twisted up and in pain. . . . When I see
patients in this kind of situation, I usually begin by asking
them some background questions about why they're here, what
their history is, how long they've been ill, and so on. The first
thing I asked her was whether she usually used a wheelchair.
Was that the way she usually got around? Apparently, even
though I thought her extremely disabled and deformed, this
was the first time she had needed to use a wheelchair. She had
somehow managed to cope with all the things that arthritis
means, get around her house, take care of her family, and do
her job, without having to resort to the symbolic state of "being
in a wheel chair." Right away, that put us in touch with each
other, and the encounter shifted to an emotional level. . . .
The illness is horrible to most people, and they never talk about
it to the patient, but it is an everyday thing to you, something
you have dealt with, something you know about, and therefore
not horrendous or awful. I could feel that between us—that
contact.

    I then moved into doing a physical assessment and looking
at her various joints. Thinking about this later, I realized one
of the ways I was able to communicate with her, really get to
some of the things she felt, was just by the way I looked at her
joints. I made distinctions about swelling, the level of inflam-
mation, and so on. It is possible to touch a person and move
the person's hand or wrist, and say: "I can tell that this must
be really painful right now," or "It looks like you haven't been
able to use this hand for a long time." (Benner & Wrubel
1989, pp. 9–10)

Hastings continued with the physical assessment of the patient, asking
her the kinds of questions she typically asked. When she finished the
examination she said to the patient,

    "Rheumatoid arthritis really has not been nice to you." She
    burst into tears, and her daughter did also, and I sat there,
    very close to losing it myself. She said: "You know, no one has

ever talked about it as a personal thing before, no one's ever talked to me as if this were a thing that mattered, a personal event." (in Benner & Wrubel, 1989, p. 11)

Understanding how such engrossment is possible is made clear in an interpretation of another example of nursing excellence by Benner & Wrubel (1989). In this case, the nurse had so vividly described a mastectomy in her preoperative teaching that her patient could not believe that she herself had not had a mastectomy. Benner & Wrubel give an insightful interpretation of the nurse's ability to imaginatively describe her patient's future experience. "She had not stood outside the patient's realm of experience in her teaching. . . . She was not the aloof health care professional standing outside the patient's community and realm of possibility. . . . Instead, she had truly stood alongside the patient, and in her teaching she had conveyed that this could happen to her too" (p. 13). True engrossment involves living through patients' experiences with them. Intersubjective knowledge gained from sharing in the lived experience of illness and treatment further enables nurses to become engrossed in their patient's experience as a "personal event . . . that mattered."

Caring, however, involves more than sharing in the patient's experience. Noddings (1984) contends that there also must be an actual motivational shift in which there is "displacement of interest from my own reality to the reality of the other." Then "we see the other's reality as a possibility for us" and "must act to eliminate the intolerable, to reduce the pain, to fulfill the need, to actualize the dream" (p. 14). Lessening the pain, meeting the need, and actualizing the dream requires us "to act as one-caring . . . with special regard for the particular person in a concrete situation. . . . The one-caring desires the well-being of the cared-for and acts to promote that well-being" (p. 24).

A caring relationship not only involves the one-caring but also the response of the one cared-for. As Noddings (1984) states succinctly, "The cared-for contributes to the caring relation . . . by receiving the efforts of one-caring, and this receiving may be accomplished by a disclosure of his own subjective experience in direct response to the one-caring or by a happy and vigorous pursuit of his own projects" (pp. 150–151).

Orlick (1988) provides an excellent example of both motivational shift by the one-caring and of the response of the one cared-for in a description of a relationship she had with her patient. During the two months in which she cared for that patient, she and the patient had developed a very close relationship. The patient was transferred to Intensive Care after surgery, and he almost died. When he was again under Orlick's care, he was unusually lethargic, expressionless, and avoided eye contact with her. Orlick described their relationship in a way that shows both her motivational shift and the patient's response.

> *I tried various therapeutic interventions that I had learned in nursing school to get him to talk about his feelings, but all he would do was nod his head or stare blankly at the wall. Finally, I said to him: "You just don't care any more, do you?" All he did was shake his head. At that point my emotions "got the best of me." I had been working with this man for two months, knew his family, and had developed a relationship with him. I felt he was shutting me out and it made me feel sad, frustrated, and angry all at once. At that moment, all the therapeutic nursing intervention strategies I had learned just left me. I responded to Gerald on a gut level. I yelled at him, "Well damn it Gerald, we care!"*

Surprised by her outburst, Orlick abruptly left her patient. Gerald was crying when she returned. When she asked him if he was alright, he responded by squeezing her hand and saying, "Thank you."

In the above example a motivational shift and response becomes evident. Orlick had cared for Gerald for two months, and he had responded by receiving and cooperating in that care. It is Orlick's frustration at her patient's refusal to accept her continued care, however, that reveals the intensity of the motivational shift. A less obvious form of motivational shift takes place when her professional care is replaced by the intense personal outburst, "Well, damn it, Gerald, we care!" Then Gerald understood that her past care and her frustration were motivated by her personal concern for him. He responds to the concern evident in her past care and in her current frustration by appreciatively accepting his future care by squeezing her hand and saying, "Thank you."

The foregoing relationship also exemplifies natural caring. Orlick obviously cares for Gerald, personally and naturally. For Noddings (1984) one should foster the well being of others out of natural caring if that is possible. If natural caring is not possible, then, according to Noddings, one should care out of the desire to be virtuous. She contends that morality is an "active virtue" that requires two feelings. First, there "is the sentiment of natural caring." Second, there is sentiment that grows out of a kind of remembrance which Saul Bellow (1989) has called "an affective recollection" (p. 3). According to Noddings, the remembrance of natural caring "sweeps over us as a feeling—as an I must—in response to the plight of the other and our conflicting desire to serve our own interests" (p. 79-80). When faced with such an inner conflict, "I have a picture of those moments in which I was cared for and in which I have cared, and I may reach toward this memory and guide my conduct by it if I wish to do so." Doing so (ethical caring) "requires an effort that is not needed in natural caring" (p. 80). Noddings identifies the ethical with that which is done out of a sense of what one ought to be. But Noddings does not elevate what ought to be over natural caring as some philosophers, such as Kant, have done. An ethic of caring "strives to maintain the caring attitude and is dependent upon, and not superior to, natural caring" (p. 80). The sentiments of natural caring and of concern with being our best self both motivate moral action. In the first case I care because I want to help others, in the latter case I care because I want to be a good person.

It is important to nursing ethics to recognize how Noddings' (1984) interpretation of the "ethical" differs from the ethical of traditional philosophy. In traditional ethics what one ought to do is determined by its coherence with moral norms, such as the utilitarian principle of the greatest happiness for the greatest number or the Kantian principle of autonomy. In contrast, for Noddings, the ethical refers to that which is done out of the desire to be a good person, that desire being informed by the experience of having been cared for. This appreciative remembrance informs the meaning of being a good person. In addition to informing the meaning of being a good person, affective recollection empowers the caregiver to make the required shift from concern for self—being a good person—to engrossment with and motivational displacement toward the person needing care.

The shift from self to others is essential in nursing care. Milton Mayerhoff (1971) contributes to Noddings' interpretation of the relationship of affective remembrance to caring. He shows how caring is evoked by its integral relationship to truth, patience, honesty, trust, humility, hope, courage (pp. 11–28), autonomy, faith, and gratitude (pp. 78–87). He defines caring as a relationship with another person that "helps him grow and actualize himself" (p. 1). Since my growth has been fostered by the care of parents, teachers, and others, giving care to others is my way of expressing gratitude for the undeserved care which I have received throughout my life. Thus, Mayerhoff's treatment of gratitude is especially pertinent to Noddings' contention that remembrance of care received evokes an imperative to care. Mayerhoff reminds nurses that "caring becomes my way of thanking for what I have received" (p. 86). In this way, gratitude for care received empowers nurses to shift from care for self to care for others.

When Noddings' (1984) ethical care out of the desire to be a good person is translated into nursing care, it means that when I cannot care for my patient out of natural caring, then I should care for him or her because I want to be a good nurse. Caring for a patient out of the desire to be a good nurse is exemplified in the care given by Elizabeth Ashton (1988) for one of her patients. Ashton described a patient named Ben, who had a paralyzing spine injury at C3 and C4, as a very demanding patient who expected immediate attention. "His demanding ways made most of us want to avoid him, even if we felt guilty about it later" (p. 21). At the end of a particularly busy shift which was very under-staffed, Ben's light was on once again. With many loose ends still to tie up before she could leave the hospital, Ashton went to answer Ben's light. He was somewhat frantic from a mucus plug which needed to be suctioned. As Ashton suctioned Ben, wiped his eyes, and gave him a drink, she avoided his eyes in order that her impatience would not be obvious to him. Ashton proceeded to the nurses' station, but on her way down the hall, she could see Ben's light was on again, and she returned to his room. Ben motioned for his mouthpiece which he used to spell out words on an alphabet board. Usually Ben's use of the mouthpiece was frustrating to both Ben and the nurses because Ben was a poor speller and the process was time consuming. Over Ashton's protests that she had to go, Ben insisted on spelling the words, "thank you." Ashton relates, "I continued looking at him, surprised and de-lighted, but my eyes suddenly welled with tears. Personal contact—that was all he'd wanted" (p. 21).

In the above example, it is obvious that Ashton did not care for Ben naturally but gave him excellent nursing care out of her desire to be a good nurse. Indeed, one has the impression that she and the other nurses were very exasperated with Ben. In spite of this exasperation, however, this type of illness made it imperative that nurses respond to his call immediately or he could suffocate. The story provides a definite impression that Ben had been exploiting the potential urgency of his situation to get attention from the nurses. Ashton's response to his second call is clearly an example of acting out of the ethical sense of caring.

The above example suggests an answer to a difficult question concerning the relationship between natural caring and ethical caring, especially in health care. Can nurses learn natural caring from ethical caring? Put differently, are acts done out of wanting to care and acts done out of a desire to be a good nurse such different forms of motivation that one could not engender the other? The above example helps us understand a possible solution to this seeming dilemma. In the above case, it is evident that Ashton's transition from caring for Ben out of the desire to be a good nurse to one of wanting to care for Ben comes in response to appreciation shown by Ben for care given. This is very apparent because of Ben's condition. All he wanted was to communicate with his nurse in a way that well people take for granted. When someone does something for us, we normally respond by thanking him or her. Due to his incapacity, Ben was unable to do this without great effort. He appreciated the good care Ashton provided and simply wanted to thank her. Note that her care was not exceptional, except that it was given on a busy night. By responding to Ben's calls, she was doing the morally good work typical of nurses who give competent care to their patients. Although her return to his room was done begrudgingly, it certainly indicated that she was willing to give extra care to her patient under difficult circumstances. However, perhaps her most significant moral activity was accepting his thanks by meeting his eyes and showing her gratitude for his appreciation. Now he had become a person, in the full meaning of that word, for whom she cared naturally. Care often moves from being ethically motivated to being naturally motivated when patients respond with gratitude for care given, and caregivers respond personally by accepting that gratitude.

In the foregoing example, good care refers both to personal morality and excellent practice at the same time. Since excellent practice aims at moral good, nurses are being moral when they practice well. Many nurses also implicitly grasp the connection between being morally good and excellent practice as evidenced in our study of fulfillment in nursing cited earlier in this book. In almost every case, fulfillment came when the moral import of excellent practice became apparent in the response of patients or their loved ones. That such care can be very technical as well is evident in the case of the nurse cited previously who described her patient as a "GCS5T, E4, M1, VT." Beyond her technical expertise, her fulfillment came from seeing the patient follow a command for the first time—"moving his thumb made me feel wonderful inside" (Bishop & Scudder, 1990, p. 99). It seems odd for anyone to find such fulfillment from a thumb being moved. The full significance of the thumb movement could only be grasped by those who see its significance in the context of health care practice. In contrast, another nurse found fulfillment in a very ordinary nursing care situation.

> The most fulfilling experience I ever had was when a child I was caring for arrested but was successfully resuscitated. I had written my notice that day—I wanted out of nursing—it was killing me. The baby stopped breathing while we were on the elevator coming back from X-Ray. I did mouth-to-mouth on her until we got back to the room and the code team arrived. The baby responded beautifully. Naturally I felt good. But when the mother praised me for "saving" her baby, I tried to tell her that what I did was not so special; anyone can do mouth-to-mouth. "But it was you," she said. "You were there. If you hadn't wanted to be a nurse in the first place and been working that day, I wouldn't have my baby." (Bishop & Scudder, 1990, p. 101)

It is significant that this nurse made her decision to continue in nursing after being made aware of the moral import of nursing practice by the appreciation of the mother of the child to whom she had given the expected routine care which did, in fact, save the baby's life.

In nursing, then, it is important to be able to recognize the moral significance of caring as it is evident in practice. When the personal sense of caring is stressed, it is easy to overlook the moral sense of practice. Noddings (1984), for example, while helping nurses to more fully grasp the meaning of caring, does not adequately grasp the moral sense of practice. This is evident in her treatment of her professional field, education. In discussing caring in education, she does not begin with the study of education but with caring. Then, after determining what caring is, she attempts to discover the form "caring takes in the teaching function" (p. 70). Perhaps the fact that she regards teaching as a function rather than as a practice accounts for her failure to recognize that the practice of teaching, like nursing, can be a concrete source for understanding the meaning of caring for others. She seems to believe that we come to a true understanding of the meaning of caring by interpreting personal caring. Then she uses her interpretation to determine what counts as caring in education. In her treatment of learning to care through practice, she simply regards practice as a source of learning caring by doing. She does not seem to grasp that caring practices can disclose the meaning of caring.

Both Gadamer (1981) and MacIntyre (1984) show how interpretation of practice can disclose how the good is fostered in the world. In nursing the good is fostered by caring. Understanding the meaning of caring is enhanced for nurses by the theories of caring of Gilligan (1980) and Noddings (1984). But for their ethic of caring to make its potential contribution to nursing, the integral relationship between caring and nursing practice must be grasped.

If this integral relationship is not recognized, personal caring and professional caring are understood as separate forms of caring. When this is the case, a nurse thinks of nursing practice and nursing ethics as being separate from each other, with nursing ethics focusing on making decisions that affect nursing care but over which nurses often have little control, such as when to pull the plug. Consequently, nurses often fail to see the moral implications of the day-to-day care over which they have almost complete control. When personal care and professional care are integrated, being a good person and being a good nurse become one, as the foregoing examples illustrate. When this integration occurs, Noddings' (1984) ethical caring takes on new meaning. When I cannot care naturally, she contends that I should care for others because I want to be a good person. In a philosophy of nursing practice, this would be translated into when I cannot care naturally for my patients, then I should care for them because I desire to be a good nurse. Being a good nurse requires me to make Noddings' motivational shift from preoccupation with myself to *concern* for the patient who needs my help. When this occurs, the two powerful motives for caring—natural caring for the other and the desire to be good (i.e., a good nurse)—become one. In nursing, as practiced, these two motives seem to belong together and to be required for excellent nursing practice. Excellent nursing requires that I care both because I am concerned for the well-being of my patients and because I want to be a good nurse. When these motives come together, the meaning of good in good nurse and good person become one.

Clearly, this common meaning of good nurse and good person often occurs in nursing practice. All the examples we have used in this chapter to illustrate Gilligan's (1980) and Noddings' (1984) interpretations of caring are the same examples we have previously used to illustrate excellent nursing practice. The fact that they were previously used without conscious reference to their moral import, but in this chapter were used as examples of caring, supports our contention that, in nursing, the practical and the moral sense of care coincide.

to become concerned that the stress on scientific technology is leading nurses to neglect nurse–patient relationships, always a significant aspect of traditional nursing. This is especially true of those nurses whose understanding of the meaning of personal has been enhanced by interpreters of the meaning of human existence. Nonetheless, an adequate articulation of contemporary nursing practice would need to show how scientific technology and personal relationships can be understood as integrally related in a caring practice.

Showing how scientific technology and the personal are actually or potentially integral in a caring practice by phenomenological interpretation contrasts sharply with holistic attempts to reconstruct the meaning of being a person after scientific analysis has torn it asunder. In nursing, one attempt to restore unity to the concept of person involves a bio-psycho-social approach. Biological, psychological, and sociological analyses, however, even when used together, do not restore unity so much as identify three distinct measures of the concept of person. In effect, this approach is an attempt to put Humpty-Dumpty back together again. Rather than such an approach, we believe that unity can best be achieved through an *integral* interpretation of caring. Our contention follows logically from our phenomenological interpretation of nursing as a caring practice. In this approach, unity is sought by following the initial phenomenological move of focusing on the things themselves as they appear in human experience before they are torn apart by scientific analysis. We do not, in fact, experience ourselves as biological beings, sociological beings, or psychological beings which we must put together by an act of will (Kockelmans, 1979, p. 22). We do, in fact, experience ourselves as concrete whole beings. Neither do we experience our world as a material world, a biological world, a psychological world, nor a sociological world but as one world. Nor do we experience ourself as separate from our world, but as we have shown through our interpretation of Heidegger (1962), the man-world relationship is one. However, self and world have been fractured and split by the various disciplines which study certain aspects of the world. These specialized ways of studying the world have made important contributions to our understanding of various aspects of the world such as disease and treatment. But when we regard these abstract academic disciplines as fundamental reality, we make the mistake that the great scientist and philosopher, Alfred North Whitehead (1925) called "misplaced concreteness." By this he meant that we tend to think of science as dealing with the concrete world when, in fact, science is a very specialized and abstract way of dealing with the world. Our immediate and initial experience of the world is what is concrete. In the phenomenological tradition, unity is not achieved by reuniting the academic disciplines in Humpty-Dumpty fashion but by returning to the unified world of lived experience from which the theoretical specialized disciplines were initially abstracted. Two ways in which abstract scientific explanation can be incorporated into the lived world without artificially reconstructing it are the hermeneutic spiral and triadic dialogue.

THE HERMENEUTIC SPIRAL

Nurses often use the hermeneutic spiral without being aware of it. This occurs when nurses begin by giving nursing care in the lived world. Then, when scientific explanation is needed to explain what was occurring in the caregiving situation, nurses apply it to the situation. Armed with this better understanding, they return to the lived world better able to give care. In phenomenological interpretation, the movement from the lived world to scientific explanation and back to the lived world is called the hermeneutic spiral (Strasser, 1985; Bishop & Scudder, 1990). The following is an excellent example of the use of the hermeneutic spiral in nursing care in which scientific technology and personal relationships are integrally related in a caring practice.

> It was a typical morning with doctors coming and going, patients going off to tests, etc., when I walked into one of my patients' rooms. A vascular surgeon and a neurosurgeon had just come out of her room. The patient was with her daughter and they were discussing the impending surgery. The patient was slowly going blind due to an aneurysm at the optic chiasma, and prior to coming to our hospital, the patient admitted her husband into an ICU in Santa Barbara with a heart attack. Under the circumstances, the patient was quite jittery—the surgery planned was a bypass of cranial arteries followed by a craniotomy to remove the aneurysm—after the pressure had been released around it.

I entered the room and asked how she was doing. Her first words were, "Should I have the surgery? Do you think it is safe?"

I replied, "You couldn't have finer surgeons than you have here and I can't make that decision for you."

She took a deep breath and began to express her many fears and concerns about the surgery. She expressed the thought that if she didn't have the surgery she would only get progressively more blind but still live. If she had the surgery she could die, she could go completely blind, she could be permanently disabled physically, or she could live with the remaining part of her vision. Instead of agreeing with her or interjecting my comments, I just kept silent. I felt that it was better to let her verbalize. After she had carried on this conversation with herself, I asked her if she would like me to explain what would be going on, to which she agreed. I took in Ichabod Crani—a plastic puzzle of the head with removal parts and identification of all the parts—brain, bone, veins, arteries, etc. In the next hour we played with the parts, and I answered her questions. By the end of the hour the patient had decided that since she had come all this way, she would go ahead with the surgery.

When I finally left the room, I felt that the patient had made the right decision but that she had made it on her own. I felt good because I had given her a very descriptive account, in terms she could understand, of what was to happen to her. I had tried to remain unbiased and open and answer her questions accordingly. It was a very positive experience and it seemed to be for her. (Benner, 1984, pp. 87–88)

The nurse in the foregoing example does not respond to her patient as a patient in general but as the person she meets—full of fears concerning surgery. She responds to the person she meets by remaining silent so as to allow the patient to express all of her fears and misgivings. When the nurse recognizes that one source of the patient's fears is lack of understanding of what is involved in her surgery, the nurse shares objective information about any brain with her patient. This dialogue, like most dialogues between nurse and patient, involves relating the personal and the impersonal. In this dialogue, although the content of the dialogue is objective, its purpose obviously is to help the patient gain a clearer understanding of what will be done to her and what will be the likely outcomes in terms of her life. It is significant that the patient's decision is made out of this dialogue with her nurse. This process is obviously very different from objective decision making in which the nurse functions as an expert supplying information as *input* into the patient's decision-making process. In contrast, in this dialogue nurse and patient consider together what will be done to the patient and what will be its likely outcome for the patient. The manner of this dialogue not only prepares the patient to make her own decision but actually empowers her to make it.

It is interesting that the decision with which nurse and patient are wrestling is usually made in the physician and patient interaction. We do not know why the patient felt an obvious need to engage in dialogue with her nurse on this matter, but we can make an educated guess. The patient probably had just engaged in a typical technical, impersonal, and brief (considering what was involved) "dialogue" with her physicians in a situation which did not foster, or possibly did not even allow, real personal dialogue. The patient probably was made to feel that she should not take the physician's valuable time with such "minor" considerations as the possible loss of her life. But the nurse, conveying to her that she was open and had time for such considerations, affords an example of the hermeneutic spiral. She begins by entering into a caring relationship with her anxious patient. Helping relieve the patient's anxiety requires her to use scientific and technological explanation. During the explanation, she relates to the patient in a way that empowers the patient to make her own decision. As a consequence of the explanation given in a caring relationship, the patient is able to make a decision she could not make when confronted with it as given in the scientific, technological explanation and attitude of her physicians.

TRIADIC DIALOGUE

In addition to the hermeneutic spiral, triadic dialogue also makes possible the inclusion of scientific technology into a personal caring relationship. Martin Buber's (1958) treatment of I-It and I-Thou relationships sets a framework for showing how triadic dialogue makes it possible to treat a diseased body in a specialized objective manner and at the same time relate to the whole person being cared for. Buber's treatment of I-It is especially appropriate to nursing care because it describes the impersonal from a technological point of view. An I-It relationship is one in which one person is detached from another, has knowledge about the other, and uses this knowledge to achieve objectives set by the user of objective knowledge. Furthermore, this relationship is onesided in that the "I" side dominates the relationship with minimal regard for the response of the other, except as it relates to the purpose of the user. An I-It relationship also is partial in that the person responded to as "It" is reduced to fit into a category, that is, the hysterectomy in Room 104; the "It" partner being only of worth as he or she responds to the wishes of the "I" partner.

To help clarify this I-It relation, we offer an example of very competent nursing when viewed from an objective point of view. In order to give the most efficient care possible, a nurse working in a cardiovascular intensive care unit garners all possible objective information about the patient drawing medical information and general information from the laboratory reports, the physician's notes, EKG strips, medical history, and nursing notes. The nurse carefully studies the textbook description of the patient's disease and how this individual patient fits the generalized category. The nurse develops a careful, thorough plan of care for the patient exactly as she will follow it in giving nursing care. The plan, of course, allows the minor adjustments which changing contingent factors may require. The nurse positively reinforces the patient with smiles and token rewards when the patient conforms to the plan. In short, he or she is a model of technological efficiency in nursing.

Buber's (1958) description of an I-Thou relationship contrasts sharply with the efficient I-It relationship as presented above. For Buber, the prime quality of an I-Thou relationship is mutuality, meaning that both partners respond and relate to each other as persons. Furthermore, both partners are present to each other, meaning that the mutual response is to the person as encountered in a specific relationship. The person encountered has intrinsic worth regardless of usefulness to either partner. The person is not subsumed under any category (disease) or role (the patient) but is related to as a particular person. This, of course, means that the person is met as a whole person and not as a partial person defined by a role, a category, or a use.

Buber helps us to distinguish the difference between personal relationships and impersonal relationships, especially those structured by technological interventions. Unfortunately, Buber's analysis makes it difficult, if not impossible, to relate the personal and impersonal. For example, an I-Thou relationship which clearly shows how the personal and the impersonal are integrally related in nursing care was given in the foregoing relationship between nurse and patient. Here, scientific explanation was incorporated into a caring relationship that empowered the patient to decide about brain surgery. Although this relationship was personal in Buber's sense of the term, it was not the dyadic dialogue advocated by Buber which focuses on the relationship of the participants to each other. Instead of being dyadic, it involved a third term constituting a triad. Paulo Friere (1968) well describes triadic dialogue. "Dialogue is the encounter between men, mediated by the world," consequently it does not involve just two persons (A and B) but "rather 'A' with 'B', mediated by the world" (p. 76, p. 82). In triadic dialogue, two persons discuss the meaning of something in the world with each other. Triadic dialogue is constituted by the relationship of the two partners to the event in the world, as well as their relationship to each other (Scudder & Mickunas, 1985, pp. 33–57; Bishop & Scudder, 1990, pp. 152–161). In the above example, the event being discussed is the nature and meaning of the proposed operation. Note that the triadic structure of this dialogue makes it possible for the nurse to talk objectively about the brain and the forthcoming operation but at the same time to be personally related to her patient. In addition, a triadic dialogue makes it possible for the partners in an I-Thou relationship to have an end beyond the relationship itself. In Buber's interpretation, a true I-Thou relationship has no end beyond itself. It is an end in itself. Friends are together merely because they want to be together; they enjoy being in the presence of each other. The nurse in the above relationship was not with the patient primarily because she wanted to be or enjoyed being with this particular person but in order to give nursing care. In other words, most dialogues in nursing care have ends beyond themselves; fostering the well being of patients. For this reason, nurses usually engage in triadic dialogue rather than the dyadic dialogue proposed by Buber. Such dialogues are triadic because they are constituted not only by the two partners in the dialogue but also by the activities concerned with fostering the well-being of the

patient. In the above example, the nurse interjects objective information about the brain into the dialogue because it helps accomplish the
goal of nursing care—the patient's well being.

Triadic dialogue involves two integral relationships on the part of
the nurse and the patient. One relationship is obviously with the other
person and involves concern for that person as he or she is encountered in the meeting. The other relationship is with something in the
world, which often must be treated objectively, such as the brain to be
understood. But in the nursing relationship, this in-the-world aspect of
the dialogue is often missed because the discussion concerns the body
of one of the partners. But note how, in the above example, the brain
of the other person is treated objectively as any human brain in the
world in a way that helps a particular patient understand what will be
done to her brain and, more importantly, what the likely consequences
will be for her life.

Nurses not only must treat the body as an object when communicating with patients but also when communicating with other health care
workers. This is very apparent in charting.

10 A.M.	*77 y.o. white female admitted to room 604 with chief complaint of burning on urination. T. 101° P. 92 R. 24. B/P 138/84. Face flushed and dry. Yellowish-green bruise, 2 inches in diameter, noted on left hip. Wears dentures. Unable to obtain urine specimen.*
11 A.M.	*Urine specimen to laboratory (50 cc.) Urine cloudy and dark yellow. Forced fluids. Water 200 cc.*
12 noon	*Refused lunch. Gingerale 150 cc.*
1 P.M.	*Water 200 cc.*
1:30 P.M.	*Voided 350cc. Urine cloudy and dark yellow.*
2 P.M.	*Coke 100 cc.*
3 P.M.	*T. 100 P. 88 R. 22. Skin remains dry but no longer flushed.*

In charting, nurses treat the patient as anybody by treating the patient's
body as any body. In impersonal description, such as charting, nurses
reduce patients to objects. Consequently, they can easily forget that

these vital signs and statistics about fluid intake and urinary output are those of a particular person. She could be a grandmother whose eyes light up when they meet the face of her granddaughter and who, when holding her tenderly to her breast, forgets her boredom and pain.

When nurses treat patients impersonally, they must always remember that they are dealing with persons. Persons are entitled to the rights and respect due a person. This, of course, is very important for those who regard the nurse as a patient advocate. One meaning of such advocacy is ensuring that patients are given their rights. A second meaning is that nurses must help particular patients find personal meaning in their illness and treatment. This requires nurses to engage in personal relationships with patients. Remember how Ashton (1988) responded with personal appreciation when Ben wrote with great difficulty, "Thank you."

When nurses engage in such mechanical routines as charting, efficient and accurate impersonal recording of information is absolutely necessary. Buber (1958) is right when he says "without It man cannot live." But he is also right when he says, "He who lives with It alone is not a man" (p. 34). It is true that nurses must engage in many impersonal relationships, but the nurse who always remains in I-It relationships never encounters persons and thus misses that relationship that identifies us as human beings.

Triadic dialogue is a way of being that can incorporate a scientific, technological way of being with the body object within a caring, personal relationship between nurse and patient. Thus, it describes a way of being that meets Gadow's (1985) contention that nurses must be able to attend the body object without reducing the patient to the status of an object (pp. 33–34). Triadic dialogue is a human relationship through which nurse and patient are able to care for the body object together.

CARING FOR THOSE SUFFERING
FROM INTERVENTION

It has become more difficult for nurses to relate to patients personally due to the increased use of medical technological interventions in patient care. Before the advent of these interventions, the need for nursing primarily came from illness. Now nursing care often is required due to injury incurred by interventions. The following narrative describing a person suffering from both cancer and interventions was given at a regional nursing conference by his friend who used it as an example of why nurses must care for those injured by intervention as well as by disease.

Irv had been my friend for 50 years. He lived with cancer for over two years after the best medical prognosis gave him at best a few weeks to live. During the summer he received his death sentence, I flew up to visit him to play tennis, fish, philosophize, and reminisce about our long friendship. During the next summer before his winter death, we played tennis for the last time. Somehow he managed to beat me soundly. Given his condition at the time, he convinced me that Norman Cousins, one of his favorite authors, was right in arguing that the spirit can overcome bodily ailments. When we discussed his treatment for cancer, he constantly praised his nurse, Donna. In fact, he insisted that I send her an autographed copy of my coauthored book on the philosophy of nursing which had just been published [Bishop & Scudder, 1990]. Irv contrasted Donna with his physician who he described as a very competent intervention technology physician. His physician diagnosed and prescribed and his conversations with Irv were cryptic and technological. In contrast, Donna related to him primarily as a fellow human being. Of course, she dealt with medical technology. In fact, she was the one who administered the chemotherapy, related his prescriptions to him, and gave directions on how to take them. But she talked with him and touched him as a fellow human being for whom she cared. As Irv put it, "She is on my team and she brought me through." She cheerfully responded when he called to ask how to lessen the pain, how to control the diarrhea, and how to alleviate the constipation, which often were more the consequence of treatment than illness. In short, although she was involved in administering the technological intervention, she also gave the care which helped Irv bear the interventions. Her care helped the body heal and his spirit to cope with the consequences of intervention. But first and foremost, throughout the interventions,

she related to Irv as a fellow human being for whom she cared.
Irv experienced what Albert Schweitzer has called, "the terrible things that men can undergo" [Spiegelberg, 1975, p. 234].
Cancer is terrible but so are the prescribed interventions.
When those who administer the interventions do so with empathic communication and touch which affirm our common humanity, then "the terrible things that men can undergo" can be endured and on good days the spirit can revive and miracles can occur.

The Miracle

As we walked off the court, I expected an excuse from my long time doubles partner, Irv. Not that he needed an excuse; he had played well for someone in his state of health. But instead of an excuse, he commented with a twinkle in his eye, "Oh well, I have my good days." I remembered that good day—the miracle of yesterday. He had played at first as he had today. I had taken pace off the ball and hit to him so we could have a decent game. Then, in the middle of the first set, the miracle began. The fire returned to Irv's eyes, the power to his stroke, his fluid movements once again propelled him across the court, and he rushed the net wielding his racquet, as his Viking ancestors once did their axes. Big Irv was back!

What brought about this miracle? Irv had told me his secret two years before when his physician had given him weeks to live. Irv had predicted that his spirit would overcome his body and to prove it, he invited me to come to Northern Wisconsin the next summer for a week of tennis and fishing. Overcome it he did. He beat me that summer, but not as soundly as later, on that good day when the miracle occurred. Between those two summers, new and stronger interventions were prescribed. Irv had not known about the terrible interventions that he would undergo when he first made his optimistic prediction. His miracle required more than his courageous, zestful spirit; it also required the care of Donna, who not only attended to his body but who cared for Irv in a way that helped him not only live with a life-limiting illness but also with the terrible interventions used to fight his cancer. (Scudder, 1990)

Dying patients such as Irv often live in the hope of future good days. Discussions of the termination of treatment should concern not just the possibility of biological life but the possibility of good days. Care such as Donna's not only helps foster longer life but also those good days which make life worth living.

EVOCATIVE-EXPRESSIVE LANGUAGE AND PROPOSITIONAL LANGUAGE

The enthusiastic response to the foregoing presentation by the nurses at the conference surprised the presenter. He was accustomed to receiving a few polite comments from nurses about the clarity and, occasionally, the profundity of his thought. Such enthusiastic appreciation was totally unexpected. The reason for the different response was evident, however, when he reflected about his presentation. Normally his papers were written in the neutral, arid, propositional language of the academy, especially as used in science and philosophy. He had been unable to write about his friend Irv in propositional language. His love of and admiration for Irv and his appreciation of Donna called forth expressive and evocative language. Speaking in this language also expressed his admiration for caring nurses, like Donna, in a way that helped the nurses present rediscover the meaning of being a nurse.

Expressive language, the language of feeling and sensitivity, conveys our attunement to the world. Evocative language is the language that calls forth particular ways of being in the world. Expressive-evocative language is the language of personal relationships. In contrast, propositional language, the language of science and technology, is the language of detachment and analysis. Detached separation, linear progression, and if-then logic characterize our way of being in propositional language. Propositional language yields knowledge about things that can be used to control them. Expressive-evocative language is the language of involvement, concern, and connection. It can contain propositional language as was evident in our example of the nurse using Ichabod Crani to explain a proposed surgical procedure. On the other hand, propositional language excludes personal language on the grounds that it is merely subjective. Recall how Cousins (1989) was warned not to use personal, antecdotal language when talking to medical scientists. Also recall how the man dying of cancer responded to the medical scientists' dismissal of mere incidents and antecdotes by retorting that what they called a mere incident, he called his life and mere antecdotes, the story of his life.

Nursing practice requires an integral relationship between evocative-expressive and propositional language. Expressive language conveys feelings about the world, whereas evocative language calls forth some kind of action that transforms the world. In contrast, propositional language is the objective means that abstractly reorders the world in terms of some rational system. When a nurse expresses his or her concern for a patient's well being by tone of voice and therapeutic touch, this is expressive language. When a nurse assures the patient that therapy will make it possible to walk soon, he or she uses evocative language. In actual nursing practice, expressive and evocative language often are integrally related. Propositional language, on the other hand, often seems cold, detached, and unrelated to such expression and assurance. But nursing care cannot avoid propositional language because any scientific description of disease, diagnosis, and treatment involves propositional language. Therefore, nursing requires an integral language in which the propositional and expressive-evocative are integrally related to each other. (We are indebted to Jean Gebser (1985) for his interpretation of integral.)

Most of the examples of nursing care cited in this book can be used as examples of integral language. The nurse who empowered the concert pianist with the stroke to continue with her physical therapy obviously employed evocative language that also expressed her concern for the patient's well being. Less evident is her use of propositional language with its if-then logic—if you do the therapy, then your ability to use your hand will greatly increase. A striking example of the use of propositional language was the nurse who described her patient as a "GCS5T, E4, M1, VT [who] opened his eyes but [had] no movement and was trached." But her use of integral language became evident when she said, "I can't describe the sensation I felt, but to see him follow a command for the first time—moving his thumb made me feel wonderful inside." The nurse who examined the patient with rheumatoid arthritis moved, thought about, and talked about the patient's joints propositionally. But she so well expressed her feeling for the patient's condition that the patient remarked, "No one has ever talked about it as a personal thing before, no one's ever talked to me as if this were a thing that mattered, a personal event." Orlick combined inter-vention language with "Damn it, Gerald, *we* care!" Donna's care for Irv combined scientific and technological explanation with expres-sions of care for him personally that conveyed a tone of hopefulness that resonated with and enhanced Irv's buoyant and courageous spirit. Perhaps the most striking example of integral language is the case of the neurosurgical nurse who showed her openness to the anxious patient, expressed her concern for her, gave a scientific expla-nation of the brain, and a technological description of her surgery in such a way that it empowered the patient to make her own decision. In the foregoing examples, as well as others in the book, integral language is used to bring scientific explanation of various processes, the feelings of persons, and their hope for the future into one conver-sation that fosters the well being of the patient. (For a more extensive treatment of integral language in nursing, see Bishop & Scudder, 1990, pp. 161–169, and in education see Scudder & Mickunas, 1985, pp. 104–125.)

THOUGHT AND FEELING: GENDLIN

Most nurses use integral language because concrete nursing care re-quires that thought and feelings be related to each other. Eugene Gendlin (1978) has made us aware of the need to restore the integral relationship of thought and feeling. In his book, *Focusing*, he not only makes important contributions to nurses who deal with psychological well being, but he helps them to grasp the integral relationship of thought and feeling at the base of human experience.

> In focusing one pays attention to a "felt sense." . . . A felt sense is body and mind before they are split apart. . . .
> Focusing is not an invitation to drop thinking and just feel. That would leave our feelings unchanged. Focusing begins with that odd and little known "felt sense," and then we think verbally, logically, or with image forms. . . . Thinking in the usual way, alone, can be objectively true and powerful. But, when put in touch with what the body already knows and lives, it becomes vastly more powerful.

Truth does not lie in thought alone. It lies in how various thoughts relate to experience. . . . Experience can never be equated with concepts. But experience is not "undefined" either. It is more organized, more finely faceted by far, than any concepts can be. And yet it is always again able to be lived further in a new creation of meaning that takes account of, and also shifts, all the earlier meanings. (pp. 165–166)

Nurses often understand what is happening to their patients by the felt sense of the meaning of a given situation. Many disagreements between physicians and nurses result from the difference between the integral way of thinking of nurses and the objective, conceptual thinking of physicians as the following example illustrates.

We had a patient who had an esophageal dilatation in X-Ray. She was a very uncomplaining woman of about 60 years of age. When she came back her vital signs were OK, and she was up in the bathroom. Later she started getting nauseated and she had streaks of very light pink drainage which I could account for by dilatation procedures, but I just had this feeling that something else was going on. She became worse; she became very nauseated. I called the house officer to check her. The house officer examined her but was not ordering any tests. I wanted to order blood work. I pointed out that the patient's nail beds were cyanotic. The house officer was unimpressed. It was almost time for me to go off duty when the patient started having chills with a temperature, so I called the house officer again and said there was something going on with this patient, and that I wanted to see something done for her before I went off duty. Later I found that the patient had a rupture in her esophagus; she also had aspiration pneumonia. Her pulse had gone up to 150. The house officer credited my persistence in getting early treatment in making a difference in the patient's outcome. (Benner, 1984, pp. 100–101)

Notice that in the foregoing case the nurse "had this feeling that something else was going on." The difference between the nurse's diagnosis and the physician's diagnosis is so striking that the physician did not recognize the significance of the nurse's felt sense of an impending crisis in the patient's condition. One can almost hear the physician muttering under his breath the first time he is called. "My time is being wasted by this nurse who thinks she is a physician, but who makes diagnosis based on feelings. No objective criteria for her absurd suspicions. Sure the patient's nails are cyanotic, but she is basing her request for more tests on her feelings. How like a woman!" Actually, her feelings constitute a pre-thematic awareness of impending crisis, born of years of intersubjective experience with patients when their condition was rapidly deteriorating. Such pre-thematic awareness cannot be objectively stated and precisely placed in a taxonomy, because it is the felt sense of something being wrong that precedes the objective diagnosis. Significantly, the physician responds only after the nurse supplies other objective symptoms—chills and fever—and then only after the nurse doggedly refuses to leave until further testing is done. With further testing, the medical diagnosis of a ruptured esophagus is made. In contrast, her nursing diagnosis was based on a felt sense that something is terribly wrong with this patient, requiring immediate medical attention. Her diagnosis did require some scientific technological knowledge. Nonetheless, she obviously did not come to the conclusion that something was wrong with the patient by applying science to her situation. She had a felt sense that something was going wrong.

Health care itself is initiated by a felt sense. A person's felt sense that something is wrong with his or her being in the world usually brings the person to a physician for medical diagnosis. Most medical diagnosis begins with the physician listening to the patient express that felt sense of wrongness. One of the marks of a good diagnostician is the ability to draw out and expand on the patient's felt sense of the illness in a way that facilitates diagnosis of illness as a disease.

The actual confirmation that illness is a particular disease often is done through scientific technology. Stress on scientific technology has led to focusing on disease and neglecting illness. This is an odd reversal of events in the day-to-day world. Usually, it is the experience of illness that leads a person to a physician in order to have it designated as disease so that it can be treated and hopefully cured. Illness names an experience people undergo; disease names abstract definitions of illness in terms of cause and effect. The purpose of designating illness as disease is to discover the cause of the experience of illness and to prescribe interventions that destroy or lessen the effect of disease. But the purpose of intervention in disease is to alter present or future experience of illness.

The experience of illness has been described phenomenologically as a rupture in the man-world relationship which focuses on the lived body (Gadow, 1982; Rawlinson, 1982). "Illness obstructs our ordinary access to the world and presents the body as a signifier for the way in which we are limited and can be impeded in our encounter with the world" (Rawlinson, 1982). Rawlinson contends that in illness the body does not function as it is normally expected to function. It "seems unreliable and unpredictable" (p. 75) and it becomes uppermost in the mind. In addition, illness

> results in a surrender of one's autonomy and integrity of person out of necessity or in hope that this surrender will be in the end useful in the effort to recover those capacities which the illness obstructs and threatens. This surrender makes one vulnerable and leaves one at the mercy of others in significant ways. (p. 77)

The primary reason one is willing to become vulnerable to and at the mercy of health care workers is to recover from illness and not so that health care workers can intervene in the natural history of disease. People become concerned about disease and seek help through interventions in order to avoid the experience of illness. Illness is recognized through a felt sense that something is wrong with our being-in-the-world.

Diagnosis of illness as disease often does require use of scientific technology which separates thought from feeling. When the meaning of the diagnosis is shared with anxious patients, however, physicians who really care for their patients will engage in dialogue with them out of a felt sense. Likewise, when nurses give care out of the felt sense, feeling and thought are integrally related. The *sense* in felt sense means that what is felt is intelligible—it literally makes sense. Thus, the meaning of *care* in health care refers not to an irrational inner feeling but to the felt sense that makes care for patients/clients possible and intelligible. This meaning is shared with others through dialogue in the integral language that unites the scientific and the personal.

6

Nursing:
The Practice of Caring

We have articulated nursing as a caring practice by the phenomenological interpretation of the way of nursing as practiced. Ricoeur's
(1977) description of phenomenology as philosophy that focuses on
meaning, gives meaning in terms of essence, and discloses essence
through a well-chosen example has been used to articulate nursing. We
also have used interpretation to disclose further meaning. It seems
appropriate, therefore, to conclude with a phenomenological interpretation of an example of nursing care that discloses the meaning of
nursing practice as we have articulated it in this book.

NURSING AS THE PRACTICE OF CARING:
AN EXEMPLAR

Morris Magnan (1989), a registered nurse taking his public health
course in a BSN program, was assigned to Mrs. Clark, a 76-year-old
black woman who was insulin-dependent, had congestive heart failure,
and had been bedridden for seven years. Mrs. Clark was being taken
care of by an 11-year-old granddaughter, and they lived in very poor
housing. Mrs. Clark had not been very receptive to Magnan's first
visit, which ended "almost before it began" (p. 219). But Magnan had

95

persisted and Mrs. Clark had agreed to let him visit "three times a week for thirty minutes to check her vital signs and measure her ankles" (p. 220). After Magnan completed his first assessment, which took about five minutes, he sat down "on a pile of newspapers to listen to my 'case study'" (p. 220). Mrs. Clark told him that there was no need for him to just sit around, but he told her he would remain until their 30 minutes was up. It took two weeks before Mrs. Clark stopped trying to "shoo" him away, but Mrs. Clark finally began telling him stories about her earlier life. On a subsequent visit, Mrs. Clark's sister met him at the door, stating that Mrs. Clark had refused to be bathed and would not eat. Mrs. Clark cursed at Magnan when he tried to take her blood pressure, and she smacked his hand when he touched her cheek. But he was convinced from her cold, clammy skin that she was having an insulin reaction. When Mrs. Clark recovered from the insulin shock, she apologized for her behavior to both her sister and the nurse. Magnan seized the opportunity to begin some patient teaching and arranged to meet with Mrs. Clark and her sister again the following day. Mrs. Clark was surprised to find that "feeling 'woozy, jittery, mean, and cold all over' was her way of manifesting hypoglycemia. All along she'd thought she was possessed by a demon" (p. 220).

Magnan attempted to discover the foods that Mrs. Clark liked before he started any dietary teaching. He related, "I was supposed to sort the homemade masterpieces (wetbread and grits, honey and corn muffins, buttermilk and kneebones, fried chicken and greens) into food groups and estimate calories. How would I know how many calories are in a kneebone?" (p. 220-221). Magnan continued to be puzzled as to why Mrs. Clark was bedridden until a granddaughter one day whispered the family secret. Mrs. Clark had not been out of bed since the day the police had told her that her grandson had been killed. On a visit one day, Magnan said to Mrs. Clark, "Tell me about your grandson. . . . It doesn't matter who told me, Mrs. Clark. I know. I also know you loved him very much and that's what I want to hear about'" (p. 221). Mrs. Clark "cried and talked and remembered. The air was thick with grief—and healing" (p. 221). On the next visit, Mrs. Clark began weight-bearing exercises and on Magnan's last visit, she "pulled herself up with the walker, shuffled through the most magnificent pivot I'd ever seen, and sat down in her chair" (p. 221).

The above is an example of excellent nursing care, but it is not, however, an extraordinary one. Magnan's care of Mrs. Clark would be recognized as regular nursing practice by anyone who has ever practiced in a community setting. Any experienced nurse would take the extra time required to develop the trusting relationship needed to work with a recalcitrant patient who had multiple health problems and could benefit from nursing care. The excellence of Magnan's care stems not from its uniqueness but from its quality.

Good care requires appropriated sound practice that is appropriate to a particular person's way of being. A nurse has appropriated a practice when he or she makes it his or her own. Obviously, Magnan (1989) had appropriated sound nursing practice and used it appropriately with a particular person and in a certain situation. That Magnan had appropriated the practice of nursing is evident in the way he recognized the insulin reaction, taught Mrs. Clark about her diabetes and how to control it, helped Mrs. Clark to regain her ability to walk with exercises and the use of the walker, and his recognition that good care required development of a trusting relationship. That he had personally appropriated these aspects of general nursing practice is evident in the way he has made them his own and incorporated them naturally into his relationship with Mrs. Clark. That his care is appropriate to her is evident in his attempt to deal with food which was foreign to him, in his waiting for this very recalcitrant patient to open up, in his recognition that her immobility was caused by something other than her physical illness, and in the way his concern for her extended beyond the physical care which might make walking possible to treating her grief in a manner that made walking desirable. But Magnan shared in Mrs. Clark's grief not merely in order to get her to walk but because of his concern for her as a person.

Magnan (1989) relates to Mrs. Clark as the person who is present to him in a certain situation. He is definitely not *the nurse* treating *the patient*. His excellent nursing care is personal in the true sense of that word. His caring is not that inner, beneficent, generalized feeling detached from the world which so often masquerades as caring. His concern is for the well being of the particular person who is his patient. All excellent nursing is personal in the sense that it involves relating to particular persons and giving them appropriate care. Such care does, however, sometimes require impersonal procedures and relationships designed for certain specific purposes. For example, Magnan undoubtedly recognized the insulin shock by the symptoms common to anyone experiencing insulin shock, and the exercises for weight bearing that he prescribed are those given to any patient in Mrs. Clark's condition. But his relationship to her was a person to person relationship. He respected her right to privacy by not threatening to withdraw treatment from her when she did not cooperate with his plan of care. He became personally involved in helping her grieve for her lost grandson. In short, although he used some knowledge and methods appropriate to anybody, he did not relate to any body but to Mrs. Clark.

Magnan's (1989) feelings are not separated from his thoughts in his care of Mrs. Clark. If he regarded nursing as an applied science, he would separate thought from feeling. The television advertisement cited in chapter four, which attempts to associate nursing with science and disassociate it from caring, is an excellent example of this separation. In that advertisement, feeling is associated with care and the practice of nursing is obviously derived from science. After all, the "smarts" needed by nurses is that required to pass science courses. Science itself is a theoretical study that applies to any body, therefore in nursing care, to anybody. But the care that Magnan gave was not to anybody but to Mrs. Clark. Obviously, in his recognition and treatment of insulin shock, Magnan showed that he possessed some knowledge of science. He recognized that Mrs. Clark was in insulin shock by applying scientific theory to her particular case. He also was able to recognize insulin shock because he had encountered it often before in his nursing practice. Her cold, clammy skin and her feeling jittery and cold all over are common symptoms of hypoglycemia that any competent nurse would recognize. The cursing of other persons, however, is not ordinarily a recognizable symptom of hypoglycemia. Magnan put it well when he stated that being "mean" was her way of manifesting hypoglycemia. Magnan's care for the patient incorporated the impersonal knowledge of science with his personal knowledge of Mrs. Clark. In addition, his care drew on both his knowledge of the classical symptoms of insulin shock and his previous experience of patients' responses to hypoglycemia. Often it is said that practitioners such as Magnan have a "real feel" for what they do. In chapter five, we have shown how nurses often rely on this felt sense in practice, a sense that involves an integral relationship between body and mind and between feeling and thought.

Magnan's (1989) care was evident both in his empathically entering into the experience of Mrs. Clark and in his scientific explanation to her. He did not respond to Mrs. Clark as an irrational unscientific person because she believed in demonic possession, but he did help her to understand the scientific reasons for her aggressive behavior. His care was evident in his grasp of how psychological well being affected the physical well being of Mrs. Clark. But his care was most evident in how he appropriated the practice of nursing in ways appropriate to his particular caring for this particular patient.

The care given by Magnan was obviously well selected by Benner as an exemplar of excellent practice. As the foregoing interpretation indicates, he had appropriated the practice of nursing, made it his own, and used it creatively in the care of a particular person. His creative care is a consequence of his capacity for seeing possibilities for better care. By realizing such possibilities for better care, he is actually improving his practice, and if he shares them with other nurses he also is improving nursing care. Advances in nursing practice come not only from macro reforms in nursing but from micro improvements in which one nurse shares what he or she has learned with others. Such improvement is not an end in itself but is sought to foster the physical and psychological well being of patients. Obviously, this was the goal of Magnan's excellent and innovative care of Mrs. Clark. Consequently, it fits well the definition of a practice given by Gadamer (1981) and the way in which practices are improved as described by MacIntyre (1984).

Since Magnan (1989) is working in community health, he better fits an interpretation of practice in which the legitimate authority of the nurse is exercised with minimum interaction with other health care persons than the in-between stance of the nurse, which is much more evident in hospital settings. However, we must remember that the in-between refers primarily to the web of connection through which care is given. This web of caring in community health usually refers more to the family and community than to the physicians and bureaucrats of hospital settings. Magnan, like most community health nurses, probably has to work with physicians who give medical care and under the direction of whomever is in charge of community health. However, the primary web of caring connection within which he worked with Mrs. Clark was the family. He became so enmeshed in that web that the granddaughter in the family shared with him the family secret— the dead grandson. It was through this web of connection that he was able to foster Mrs. Clark's well being and eventually her mobility.

Magnan (1989) was obviously an existential advocate for Mrs. Clark. He helped Mrs. Clark grieve for her grandson and, in so doing, helped

restore her desire to walk. He helped her understand that her irrational, antagonistic behavior was not caused by demons but by her
hypoglycemia. By entering into her lived world, he taught her a diet
that would help her control her diabetes and that was appropriate to
her lifestyle. In short, he helped her find personal meaning in her care
and treatment. His existential advocacy here was authentic care, in that
it helped her care for herself.

From Magnan's (1989) narrative of the care he gave, however, it is
difficult to know his actual motivation. From the story, he seemed to
care for Mrs. Clark at first out of a desire to be a good nurse. As he
waited for her to respond to his care and for her to share stories with
him, his care gradually became natural caring. Certainly, at the end of
their relationship, he was acting out of natural care. Irregardless of
whether his care was motivated by ethical caring or natural caring, his
care evidenced a motivational shift from his own interest to that of
Mrs. Clark. Thus, the care he gave fits Noddings' (1984) definition of
care. However, it goes beyond Noddings' definition in that one could
come to know the meaning of caring by interpreting nursing care as it
was evident in his practice.

Magnan (1989) incorporated scientific technology into a caring practice that was personal, both in that it responded to Mrs. Clark personally and in that his response expressed his personality. He was able to
incorporate the scientific technology necessary into a caring practice
that was personal because, although he was not consciously aware of it,
he used both the hermeneutical spiral and triadic dialogue. This is
evident by way of his scientific explanation that begins and ends with
giving care to a particular patient. When her situation called for it, he
used scientific understanding to diagnose her condition as hypoglycemia. By engaging in dialogue with Mrs. Clark, he came to understand her personal diet and through dialogue helped her adapt her diet
to one that was medically appropriate for her condition. He used personal dialogue together with scientific theory to discover the reason for
her inability to walk. As a result of his personal involvement with her,
he found out that she had not walked since the death of her grandson.
His understanding of certain psychiatric theories was used to explain
why she could not walk. In teaching her to walk, he undoubtedly drew
on techniques from physical therapy. In all of these examples, his use of
scientific technology usually begins with and ends in a caring practice
and is incorporated in personal dialogue.

As the foregoing paragraphs indicate, Magnan (1989) used integral language in his dialogue with Mrs. Clark. He expressed his concern for Mrs. Clark; he evoked her willingness to care for herself, including learning to walk; and he used scientific language to diagnose her condition. Rather than alternating between expressive-evocative and propositional discourse, both were integrally related in his ongoing dialogue with her. His use of integral language and the integral relation of the technology and the personal in his care all indicate that he did not separate thought from feeling in his caring practice.

Our interpretation of Magnan's (1989) care as an exemplar of excellent practice illustrates how phenomenological interpretation discloses meaning. It attempts to disclose meaning as essence through interpretation of well-chosen examples taken from actual practice.

IMPLICATIONS FOR THE NEW CURRICULUM

Disclosure of the essence of nursing as the practice of caring through phenomenological interpretation of actual nursing practice seems appropriate to the approach to nursing education called the new curriculum. Proponents of the new curriculum believe that education should foster understanding of nursing by interpretation of its meaning from within clinical situations (Moccia, 1990; Diekelmann, 1990). They reject the Tyler or technological model of education (Diekelmann, 1988; Bevis & Watson, 1989) in which students learn theory and related skills in schools of nursing and apply them later in actual situations. They also oppose its technological structure of nursing education with fixed objectives to be accomplished by certain procedures and content that are assessed in terms of the achievement of the fixed objectives.

It is not our purpose, especially in the closing chapter, to treat the new curriculum. That has been done elsewhere (Bevis & Watson, 1989; Moccia, 1990; Diekelmann, 1990; Allen, 1990; Tanner, 1990). Instead, we will simply indicate how our interpretation of the discipline and practice of nursing as disclosure of meaning from actual practice is well suited to the new curriculum by showing its appropriateness to the approach of one of its proponents, Nancy Diekelmann.

Diekelmann treats curriculum as dialogue and meaning. Curriculum thus grows out of a dialogue between faculty, practitioners, and students concerning the meaning of nursing practice. She points out that clinical "knowledge is not . . . taught by the practitioners or the clinical faculty, because clinical knowledge cannot be taught; it can only be demonstrated . . . and it can only be acquired through experience" (Diekelmann, 1988, p. 146). Although clinical knowledge cannot be taught theoretically, the meaning of practice can be articulated by practitioners, clinical faculty, and students as they dialogically interpret the clinical situations in which they participate. In this way, practice is "theory-generating," and it "is through practice that theories are refined, elaborated, and challenged" (p. 147). Articulating practice in terms of meaning is learned by students through dialogue with clinical faculty and practitioners. Dialogue as "joint reflection on a phenomenon" deepens the experience "of all participants" by disclosing the meaning of practice (p. 145). Obviously, Diekelmann's approach calls for dialogical participant interpretation of the meaning of being a nurse. Our interpretation of triadic dialogue as mutual disclosure of the meaning of specific clinical situations seems specifically suited to Diekelmann's approach. The importance of disclosure through triadic dialogical interpretation is not confined to pedagogy, however. It involves those engaged in nursing education in a much larger project, namely, disclosing the meaning of that way of being in the world called nursing. Disclosure of the meaning of that way of being as the practice of caring through phenomenological interpretation of nursing as practiced has been attempted in this book. Significantly, this specific disclosure of meaning has grown out of an ongoing triadic dialogue between a nurse and a philosopher concerning the meaning of nursing.

DEVELOPING THE DISCIPLINE OF NURSING THROUGH PHENOMENOLOGICAL INTERPRETATION

We have contended that the discipline of nursing can be developed through disclosure of the meaning of nursing as practiced through phenomenological interpretation. We have used Benner's (1984) and our (1990) own treatments of the meaning of nursing to show how direct interpretation of practice can contribute to the discipline of nursing. Benner, by disclosing excellences through narratives and their interpretation, establishes domains of legitimate authority in nursing. We show how nursing also is constituted by a unique in-between stance that is necessary for day-to-day care and is a privileged position for fostering ethical decisions made by health care teams. In addition, we have shown how nursing can be interpreted in light of various philosophical treatments of the meaning of human existence. Such use of philosophy should not be misconstrued as importing theories into nursing practice, thus contradicting our contention that nursing theory should come from the articulation of practice. Developing nursing theory from articulation of practice does not imply that nursing is sealed off from other human endeavors. One productive approach to understanding the relationship of nursing to other human endeavors is to examine nursing practice in light of philosophical interpretations of the meaning of human existence. The purpose of such interpretation is enlightenment of practitioners rather than prescription of practice. We have provided examples of how philosophical interpretations can assist in enlightening nursing practice. Gadow's (1980) interpretation of nursing as existential advocacy suggests a possible new direction for nursing. Interpreting nursing in light of the philosophies of caring of Heidegger (1962), Gilligan (1980), and Noddings (1984) indicates that nursing is a special way in which human care for the ill and debilitated is extended and enhanced. Our interpretation also indicates that nursing care, like other forms of care, involves engrossment with and motivational shift toward others so that they are concretely cared for in a web of connection. The web of connection in which nursing care is given includes a community of care called nursing. The care of this community for patients/clients can best be designated as a practice when nursing is interpreted in light of the philosophies of practice of Gadamer (1981) and MacIntyre (1984). Nursing, like all practices, grows out of a historically developed way of fostering human good in which the *way* is integrally related to the *good*. This traditional practice becomes a caring practice when it is creatively appropriated by those caring in ways appropriate to those cared for in their particular situation. Such care is continually developed and enhanced through ongoing realization of its inherent possibilities.

THE INTEGRAL RELATIONSHIP
OF DISCIPLINE AND PRACTICE

Interpreting nursing by articulating practice directly or with the help of philosophers challenges the separation of theory and practice that has fractured our world. In nursing, as we have previously shown, much of this separation has come from borrowing theories from the natural or behavioral sciences that treat the world objectively. Theories from disciplines that use the non-human to explain the human reduce human being to natural behavior and, thus, divorce theory from those practices concerned primarily with fostering human good. In contrast, when theory articulates practice, there is no separation between theory and practice. When this approach is followed in nursing, the discipline of nursing and the practice of nursing are integrally related. The discipline of nursing develops theory by articulating practice in a way that enlightens rather than dictates practice. This enlightenment, which comes from understanding the context of meaning that informs nursing practice, makes it possible for nurses to innovatively give nursing care in a way that fosters the well being of patients, nurses, and of the practice itself.

Having practicing nurses lead in the reform of nursing practice runs counter to a major trend in our culture. Our culture tends to separate thinking, doing, and feeling from each other. Following this disunity, nursing has looked to academic nurses for thinking, to practicing nurses for doing, and to caring nurses for feeling and moral concern. Those who separate thought from doing look to nursing scholars to reform nursing practice through theory development. But interpreting nursing as caring practice implies that excellent practitioners are those who should reform nursing practice. Enlightened reform, however, requires the understanding of the meaning of nursing that scholars can bring to practice. Dialogue between scholars and practitioners unites thinking and doing in a shared thoughtful practice. Reform of nursing comes primarily from practicing nurses who, enlightened by scholars, innovatively contribute to nursing practice by realizing its inherent possibilities for fostering the good. In so doing, they make apparent the integral relationship between past achievement and future advancement and between scholarship and practice.

The separation of thought from doing fosters the separation of knowledge and morality so common in our world. As we have attempted to show in previous chapters, knowledge is integrally related to morality in caring practices. Caring practices are designed to achieve a moral good, and the primary purpose of the practitioner is to foster that good. In the case of nursing, knowledge of how to practice, including theory, shows nurses how to foster the physical and psychological well being of patients/clients. We have illustrated this by showing that the same examples of excellent practice could be used to illustrate how nurses fulfill the moral imperative to care. In addition, we have shown that Benner's (1984) competencies are actual descriptions of how nurses foster the good. Since excellent practice fosters human good, the primary moral responsibility of the nurse is excellent practice.

THE INTEGRAL RELATIONSHIP
OF PRACTICE AND CARING

Those who separate doing from feeling identify caring with feeling. Rather than referring primarily to inner feeling, care names a way of being with others in which feeling and doing are integrally related. Missing this integral relationship fosters such comments as: "Jane Smith is a caring person but an incompetent nurse." But does it make sense to call a nurse a caring person who, by practicing incompetently, denies her patients the well being that nursing is designed to foster? Also when doing is separated from caring, competent nurses are believed to become caring persons by giving "extra" personal care not required by nursing practice. When nursing is understood, however, as the practice of caring, care and practice are integrally related in the relationship of nurse and patient. Thus, nurses who practice well experience being a good nurse and a caring person as one. In caring practice, good practice requires excellent, rather than "extra," care.

Excellent care comes from the unity of thought and feeling. Taking care of others requires sensitive involvement with others in webs of relationship. It involves engrossment in their way of being and motivational shift that fosters their well being with concrete action. Such care requires unified thought and feeling, regardless of whether it originates in natural caring or ethical caring. Ethical caring requires understanding the meaning of being a good person, informed and empowered by feel-ings of having been cared for by others. When being a good person is translated into being a good nurse, good nursing requires caring for the well being of others out of an understanding of the meaning of good practice, informed and empowered by concern for the physical and psychological well being of others.

Interpreting nursing as a caring practice challenges the artificial separation of practice from concern for others. This separation leads to questions such as, "Must I really care for all patients for whom I am responsible in my practice?" Obviously, this question implies that car-ing is an inner feeling unrelated to practice. Those who follow this bifurcation denigrate care by limiting it to an inner feeling of concern and hence can make statements such as, "After all, anyone can care." If it is, in fact, true that anyone can care, such care certainly is not nursing care. The caring of nurses refers to concern made concrete through practice enmeshed in a complex, intricate system of meaning. Nursing, then, is concrete care empowered by concern for the well being of each patient and craftsmanship oriented by a system of mean-ing developed to foster better health. Thus, the two meanings of care—concern for and taking care of—are one. And furthermore, caring and practice are one because practice is the way through which nurses care. In short, nursing is the practice of caring!

References

Allen, D. (1990). The curriculum revolution: Radical re-visioning of nursing education. *Journal of Nursing Education 29*, 312–316.

Aristotle. Metaphysics. Book I. (W. O. Ross, trans.). In McKeon, R. (ed.). (1941). *The basic works of Aristotle*. New York: Random House.

Arrington, D. T., & Walborn, K. S. (1989). The comfort care-giver concept. *Caring*, 24–27.

Ashton, E. (1988). A simple message. *Nursing Life, 8*(2), 21.

Bellow, S. (1989). *The bellarosa connection*. New York: Penguin Books.

Benner, P. (1984). *From novice to expert: Excellence and power in clinical nursing practice*. Menlo Park, CA: Addison-Wesley.

Benner, P. (1987). Personal communication.

Benner, P., & Wrubel, J. (1989). *The primacy of caring: Stress and coping in health and disease*. Menlo Park, CA: Addison-Wesley.

Bevis, E. O., & Watson, J. (1989). *Toward a caring curriculum: A new pedagogy for nursing*. New York: National League for Nursing.

Bishop, A. H., Scudder, J. R. Jr. (Eds.). (1985). *Caring, curing, coping: Nurse, physician, patient relationships*. University, AL: University of Alabama Press.

Bishop, A. H., Scudder J. R. (1987). Nursing ethics in an age of controversy. *Advances in Nursing Science, 9*(3), 34–43.

Bishop, A. H., Scudder, J. R., Jr. (1990). *The practical, moral, and personal sense of nursing: A phenomenological philosophy of practice*. Albany, NY: State University of New York Press.

Bradhan, C. U., Dalme, F. C., Thompson, P. J. (1990). Personality traits valued by practicing nurses and measured in nursing students. *Journal of Nursing Education, 29,* 225–232.

Buber, M. (1965). *Between man and man.* New York: Macmillan Co.

Buber, M. (1958). *I and thou* (2nd ed.). (R. G. Smith, trans.). New York: Charles Scribner's Sons. (Original work published c. 1923).

Carpenito, L. J. (1989). *Nursing diagnosis: Application to clinical practice.* Philadelphia: J. B. Lippincott.

Chambliss, D. F. (1991). What can phenomenology do for nursing? *Medical Humanities Review, 5,* 72–74.

Cousins, N. (1989). *Head first: The biology of hope.* New York: E. P. Dutton.

Diekelmann, N. (1988). Curriculum revolution: A theoretical and philosophical mandate for change. In *Curriculum revolution: Mandate for change.* New York: National League for Nursing.

Diekelmann, N. (1990). Nursing education: Caring, dialogue, and practice. *Journal of Nursing Education, 29,* 300–305.

Engelhardt, T. (1985). Physicians, patients, health care institutions— and the people in between: Nurses. In A. H. Bishop & J. R. Scudder, Jr. (eds.), *Caring, curing, coping: Nurse, physician, patient relationships* (pp. 62–79). University, AL: University of Alabama Press.

Florida Nursing News. 1988.

Foulk, G. J., Keffer, M. J. (1991). The moral foundation of nursing: Yarling and McElmurry and their critics. In P. Chinn (ed.). *Anthology on caring.* (pp. 31–46). New York: National League for Nursing.

Friere, P. (1968). *Pedagogy of the oppressed.* (M. B. Ramos, trans.). New York: The Seabury Press.

Gadamer, H. G. (1981). *Reason in the age of science* (F. G. Lawrence, trans.). Cambridge, MA: MIT Press. (Original work published in 1976).

Gadow, S. (1980). Existential advocacy: Philosophical foundations of nursing. In S. Spicker & S. Gadow (eds.), *Nursing: Images and ideals: Opening dialogue with the humanities* (pp. 79–101). New York: Springer.

Gadow, S. (1982). Body and self: A dialectic. In V. Kestenbaum (ed.), *The humanity of the ill* (pp. 86–100). Knoxville, TN: University of Tennessee Press.

Gadow, S. (1985). Nurse and patient: The caring relationship. In A. H. Bishop & J. R. Scudder, Jr. (eds.), *Caring, curing, coping: Nurse, physician, patient relationships* (pp. 31–43). University, AL: University of Alabama Press.

Gebser, J. (1985). *The ever-present origin.* (N. Barstad with A. Mickunas, trans.). Athen, OH: Ohio University Press. (Original work published 1949).

Gelvin, M. (1970). *A commentary on Heidegger's "being and time."* New York: Harper Torchbooks.

Gendlin, E. T. (1978). *Focusing.* (2nd ed.). Toronto: Bantam Books.

Gilligan, C. (1980). *In a different voice: Psychological theory and women's development.* Cambridge, MA: Harvard University Press.

Gruber, M. (1989). A dialogue with excellence: The power of certainty. *American Journal of Nursing, 89,* 502–503.

Heidegger, M. (1962). *Being and time.* (J. Macquarrie & E. Robinson, trans.). New York: Harper & Row. (Original work published 1927).

Husserl, E. (1965). *Phenomenology and the crisis of philosophy.* (Q. Lauer, trans). New York: Harper & Row. (Original work published 1911).

Kockelmans, J. J. (1979). Daseinsanalysis and Freud's unconscious. *Review of Existential Psychology and Psychiatry, 16,* 21–42.

Kohlberg, L. (1958). The development of modes of thinking and choices in years 10 to 16. Ph.D. diss. University of Chicago.

Kohlberg, L. (1981). The philosophy of moral development. San Francisco: Harper & Row.

MacIntyre, A. (1984). *After virtue.* (2nd ed.). Notre Dame, IN: University of Notre Dame Press.

Magnan, M. (1989). Listening with care. *American Journal of Nursing, 89,* 219–221.

Malasanos, L. (1991, February). Letter to Schools of Nursing Accredited by National League for Nursing with Memorandum to Gloria F. Donnelly.

Mayerhoff, M. (1971). *On caring.* New York: Harper & Row.

Moccia, P. (1990). No sire, it's a revolution. *Journal of Nursing Education* 29, 307–311.

Mohanty, J. N. (1990). What is special about phenomenology of religion? *Phenomenological Inquiry* 14, 5–16.

Noddings, N. (1984). *Caring: A feminine approach to ethics and moral education.* Berkeley, CA: University of California Press.

Orlick, S. (1988). The primacy of caring. *American Journal of Nursing,* 88, 318–319.

Ortega Y Gasset, J. (1961). *History as a system and other essays towards a philosophy of history.* New York: W. W. Norton.

Pellegrino, E. (1985). The caring ethic: The relation of physician to patient. In A. H. Bishop & J. R. Scudder, Jr. (eds.), *Caring, curing, coping: Nurse, physician, patient relationships* (pp. 8–30). University, AL: University of Alabama Press.

Polkinghorne, D. (1988). *Narrative knowing and the human sciences.* Albany, NY: State University of New York Press.

Rawlinson, M. C. (1982). Medicine's discourse and the practice of medicine. In V. Kestenbaum (ed.), *The humanity of the ill* (pp. 69–85). Knoxville, TN: University of Tennessee Press.

Ricoeur, P. (1970). Freud and philosophy: An essay on interpretation. (D. Savage, trans.). New Haven, CT: Yale University Press.

Ricoeur, P. (1977). Phenomenology and the social sciences. In M. Korenbaum (ed.). *The annals of phenomenological sociology II* (pp. 145–159). Dayton, OH: Wright State University.

Scheffler, I. (1966). Philosophical models of teaching. In R. Hyman (ed.). *Contemporary thought on teaching* (pp. 173–183). Englewood Cliffs, NJ: Prentice-Hall.

Schutz, A. (1967). *The phenomenology of the social world.* (G. Walsh and F. Lehnert, trans.). Chicago: Northwestern University Press. (Original work published 1932).

Scudder, J. R. Jr. (1980, March). *William James' philosophy of higher education.* Paper presented at annual meeting of the Association of Higher Education. Washington, D.C.

Scudder, J. R. Jr. (1990, November). Paper presented at Annual Conference, District 3, Virginia Nurses' Association, Lynchburg, Virginia.

Scudder, J. R. Jr., & Bishop, A. (1985). The foundation of health care: Natural or human. *Humanistic Psychologist, 13*(3): 10-18.

Scudder, J. R. Jr., & Bishop, A. (1986). The moral sense and health care. In A.-T. Tymieniecka (ed.), *Moral sense in the communal significance of life. Volume XX. Analecta Husserliana* (pp. 125-158). Dordrecht-Boston: D. Reidel Publishing.

Scudder, J. R. Jr., & Bishop, A. (1988, May). Impressions of the experience of black teachers and nurses in the integration of schools and hospitals in Virginia. Paper presented at Annual Conference of the Society for Phenomenology and Human Sciences. Toronto, Canada.

Scudder, J. R. Jr., & Mickunas, A. (1985). *Meaning, dialogue, and enculturation: Phenomenological philosophy of education.* Washington, DC: Center for Advanced Research in Phenomenology and University Press of America.

Sheard, R. (1980). The structure of conflict in nurse-physician relations. *Supervisor Nurse, 11,* 14-15, 17-18.

Smith, H. (1965). *Condemned to meaning.* New York: Harper & Row.

Spiegelberg, H. (1975). Good fortune obligates: Albert Schweitzer's second ethical principle. *Ethics, 85,* 234.

Strasser, S. (1985). *Understanding and explanation: Basic ideas concerning the humanity of the human sciences.* Pittsburgh, PA: Duquesne University Press.

Tanner, C. (1990). Reflections on the curriculum revolution. *Journal of Nursing Education 29,* 295-299.

Tisdale, S. (1986). *The sorcerer's apprentice: Inside the modern hospital.* New York: McGraw-Hill.

Whitehead, A. N. (1925). *Science and the modern world.* New York: Macmillan, 80-81, 84-85.

Yarling, R. R., & McElmurry, B. (1986). The moral foundation of nursing. *Advances in Nursing Science 8*(2), 63-73.

Zaner, R. M. (1985). "How the hell did I get here?" Reflections on being a patient. In A. H. Bishop & J. R. Scudder, Jr. (eds.), *Caring, curing, coping: Nurse, physician, patient relationships.* University, AL: University of Alabama Press.

Zaner, R. M. (1988). *Ethics and the clinical encounter.* Englewood Cliffs, NJ: Prentice-Hall.